URINALYSIS AND BODY FLUIDS

A SELF-INSTRUCTIONAL TEXT

EDITION 2

Urinalysis and Body Fluids
A Self-Instructional Text

Edition 2

Susan King Strasinger, D.A., M.T. (A.S.C.P.)
Director
Medical Laboratory Technician Program
Northern Virginia Community College
Annandale, Virginia

Photography by:

Donna L. Canterbury, B.A., M.T. (A.S.C.P.) SH
Chief Technologist Primary Care Center
University of Virginia Medical Center
Charlottesville, Virginia

 F. A. DAVIS COMPANY • Philadelphia

Library of Congress Cataloging-in-Publication Data

Strasinger, Susan King.
    Urinalysis and body fluids.

    Includes bibliographies and index.
    1. Urine—Analysis. 2. Body fluids—Analysis. 3. Diagnosis, Laboratory. I. Title.
[DNLM: 1. Body Fluids—analysis—programmed instruction. 2. Urine—analysis—
programmed instruction.   QY 18 S897u]
RB53.S87   1989   616.07'566   88-33503
ISBN 0-8036-8102-X

To Harry, My Editor-in-Chief

PREFACE

The objective of the second edition remains unchanged from that of the first edition: to provide the reader with a concise, comprehensive, and carefully structured introduction to the analysis and clinical significance of nonblood body fluids. The enhancements to this edition are based on suggestions of readers who have made the first edition such a gratifying success.

A major change in this edition is the tripling of the number of color plates, particularly in the area of body fluids. Ninety color plates are conveniently located at the front of the text. Primary identification characteristics are included with each plate whenever appropriate.

Further changes include enhanced coverage of renal anatomy and physiology, and expanded coverage of quality control procedures. New techniques for the analysis of body fluids are introduced, and the coverage of cell counting methods has been increased. Additional charts are provided to support the presentation of key concepts. Finally, the chapter summaries are revised and the end-of-chapter reference lists extensively updated.

SKS

ACKNOWLEDGMENTS

Preparing the second edition of *Urinalysis and Body Fluids* has been a rewarding experience. I appreciate the suggestions for improvements from the many readers of the first edition, and I trust that many of you will recognize your suggestions in this updated edition.

I am deeply indebted to Donna Canterbury for allowing me access to her extensive collection of color plates and for providing her experience in the analysis of body fluids. Again, I thank Mr. Sherwood Bramley for sharing his experience in urinalysis, and Mr. Sam Yoon for working with me on the Yellow IRIS. My colleague, Dr. Gary Ballmann, and the Northern Virginia Community College MLT students provided valuable suggestions based on their classroom use of the first edition. Also, the subtle and cheerful prodding of my editor, Jean-François Vilain, kept me on schedule for this second edition.

CONTENTS

COLOR PLATES

1 INTRODUCTION TO URINALYSIS 1

LEARNING OBJECTIVES 1
HISTORY AND IMPORTANCE 1
FORMATION 2
COMPOSITION 2
VOLUME 3
SPECIMEN COLLECTION 4
TYPES OF SPECIMENS 6
GLOSSARY 9
ABBREVIATIONS 10
REFERENCES 10
STUDY QUESTIONS 11

2 FUNCTION AND DISEASES OF THE KIDNEY 13

LEARNING OBJECTIVES 13
RENAL PHYSIOLOGY 13
RENAL FUNCTION TESTS 21
TUBULAR SECRETION AND RENAL BLOOD FLOW TESTS 30
TITRATABLE ACIDITY AND URINARY AMMONIA 32
RENAL DISEASES 32
REFERENCES 36
STUDY QUESTIONS 38

3 PHYSICAL EXAMINATION OF THE URINE 42

LEARNING OBJECTIVES 42
COLOR 42
APPEARANCE 45
TURBIDITY 45
SPECIFIC GRAVITY 46
CLINICAL CORRELATIONS 49

ODOR   50
REFERENCES   50
STUDY QUESTIONS   51

4   CHEMICAL EXAMINATION OF THE URINE   54

LEARNING OBJECTIVES   54
REAGENT STRIPS   55
AUTOMATION IN URINALYSIS   59
pH   60
PROTEIN   61
GLUCOSE   64
KETONES   67
BLOOD   68
BILIRUBIN   70
UROBILINOGEN   73
NITRITE   75
SPECIFIC GRAVITY   76
LEUKOCYTES   77
REFERENCES   80
STUDY QUESTIONS   82

5   MICROSCOPIC EXAMINATION OF THE URINE: QUALITY ASSURANCE IN URINALYSIS   87

LEARNING OBJECTIVES   87
HISTORY AND SIGNIFICANCE   88
METHODOLOGY   88
SEDIMENT CONSTITUENTS   92
QUALITY ASSURANCE IN URINALYSIS   102
REFERENCES   110
STUDY QUESTIONS   112

6   SPECIAL URINALYSIS SCREENING TESTS   116

LEARNING OBJECTIVES   116
OVERFLOW VERSUS RENAL DISORDERS   117
AMINO ACID DISORDERS   119
TRYPTOPHAN METABOLISM DISORDERS   124
CYSTINE METABOLISM DISORDERS   125
PORPHYRIN DISORDERS   126
MUCOPOLYSACCHARIDE DISORDERS   128
OTHER SCREENING TESTS   129
SUMMARY   129
REFERENCES   131
STUDY QUESTIONS   133
CASE STUDIES   135

7 CEREBROSPINAL FLUID 137

LEARNING OBJECTIVES 137
FORMATION AND PHYSIOLOGY 137
SPECIMEN COLLECTION 138
CEREBROSPINAL FLUID IN THE HEMATOLOGY LABORATORY 139
CEREBROSPINAL FLUID IN THE CHEMISTRY LABORATORY 146
CEREBROSPINAL FLUID IN THE MICROBIOLOGY
  LABORATORY 150
CEREBROSPINAL FLUID IN THE SEROLOGY LABORATORY 152
TEACHING CEREBROSPINAL FLUID ANALYSIS 152
SIMULATED SPINAL FLUID (SSF) PROCEDURE 153
REFERENCES 154
STUDY QUESTIONS 155
CASE STUDIES 159

8 MISCELLANEOUS BODY FLUIDS 160

LEARNING OBJECTIVES 160
SEMINAL FLUID 161
SYNOVIAL FLUID 166
SEROUS FLUIDS 173
AMNIOTIC FLUID 180
SWEAT 183
REFERENCES 184
STUDY QUESTIONS 187

9 GASTRIC ANALYSIS 192

LEARNING OBJECTIVES 192
PHYSIOLOGY 192
SPECIMEN COLLECTION 193
OLD TITRATION PROCEDURES 193
CURRENT TITRATION PROCEDURE 193
BASAL GASTRIC ACIDITY 194
POSTSTIMULATION GASTRIC ACIDITY 194
TERMINOLOGY 196
SUMMARY 197
REFERENCES 197
STUDY QUESTIONS 197

10 FECAL ANALYSIS 199

LEARNING OBJECTIVES 199
SPECIMEN COLLECTION 199
PHYSIOLOGY 200
FECES IN THE URINALYSIS LABORATORY 200

FECES IN THE CHEMISTRY LABORATORY   203
SUMMARY   204
REFERENCES   205
STUDY QUESTIONS   206

ANSWER KEY   209

INDEX   213

List of Color Plates

1. Normal red blood cells, one white blood cell ($\times 400$).
2. Red blood cells: Crenated and dysmorphic forms ($\times 400$).
3. Yeast: Budding form aids in identification ($\times 400$).
4. Oil droplets: Notice the refractility commonly found with artifacts ($\times 400$).
5. White blood cell clump ($\times 400$).
6. White blood cells ($\times 400$).
7. Stained white blood cells and bacteria ($\times 400$).
8. White blood cells with acetic acid: Nuclear detail is enhanced by 2 percent acetic acid ($\times 400$).
9. Squamous epithelial cells: Irregularly shaped, easily identified under low power ($\times 100$).
10. Stained squamous epithelial cells ($\times 400$).
11. Transitional epithelial cells ($\times 400$).
12. Renal tubular epithelial cells: Presence of single nucleus differentiates these from WBCs ($\times 400$).
13. Renal tubular epithelial cells and white blood cells: Notice differences in size and nuclear structure ($\times 400$).
14. Renal tubular epithelial cells under phase ($\times 400$).
15. Oval fat body: Notice refractility of fat droplets ($\times 400$).
16. Hyaline casts and mucus: Low refractive index of both elements requires reduced light to prevent overlooking them. Compare the consistent form of the casts to the irregularly shaped mucus ($\times 100$).
17. Hyaline cast ($\times 400$).
18. Hyaline cast under phase ($\times 400$).
19. Convoluted hyaline cast: Notch suggests progression to waxy form ($\times 400$).
20. Red blood cell cast: Notice the presence of free red blood cells, including ghost cells ($\times 400$).

21. Stained red blood cell cast under phase (×400).
22. White blood cell and granular cast: Granules suggest white blood cell disintegration (×400).
23. Stained white blood cell cast (×400).
24. Renal tubular epithelial cell cast: Observe the surface attachment of cells to the cast matrix (×400).
25. Stained renal tubular epithelial cell cast (×400).
26. Stained renal tubular epithelial cell cast under phase (×400).
27. Coarsely granular cast with hemoglobin pigment: A comparison of red blood cells and yeast can also be made from this slide (×400).
28. Waxy cast: Notice the irregularly broken ends (×400).
29. Stained waxy cast, white blood cells, and yeast (×100).
30. Fatty cast: Observe the refractile fat droplets on the matrix surface (×400).
31. Fatty cast under phase (×400).
32. Broad granular cast (×400).
33. Stained broad granular cast (×400).
34. Mucus (×400).
35. Uric acid crystals: Notice yellow color and variety of shapes (×400).
36. Uric acid crystals, polarized (×100).
37. Calcium oxalate crystals: Notice classic "envelope" appearance (×400).
38. Oval and classic calcium oxalate crystals (×400).
39. Triple phosphate crystals: Notice classic "coffin lid" appearance (×400).
40. Amorphous material (×400).
41. Cystine crystals: Notice colorless, hexagonal plates (×400).
42. Cholesterol crystals: Notice notched corners on many plates (×100).
43. Cholesterol crystals, polarized (×100).
44. Tyrosine crystals: Yellow color suggests presence of liver disease (×400).
45. Bilirubin crystals: Observe the classic yellow color (×400).
46. Ampicillin crystals: Bundles of crystals are seen following refrigeration (×100).
47. Starch granules: Notice refractility (×400).

48. Artifact resembling waxy cast: Notice the lack of typical cast form and the refractility ($\times 400$).
49. CSF—normal lymphocytes: Some cytocentrifuge distortion of cytoplasm ($\times 1000$).
50. CSF—normal lymphocytes and monocytes ($\times 500$).
51. CSF—neutrophils: Cytoplasmic vacuoles result from cytocentrifugation ($\times 500$).
52. CSF—neutrophils with pyknotic nuclei ($\times 500$).
53. CSF—macrophages: Notice presence of large vacuoles ($\times 500$).
54. CSF—macrophages showing erythrophagocytosis ($\times 500$).
55. CSF—macrophage containing hemosiderin stained with Prussian blue ($\times 25$).
56. CSF—macrophage with large aggregated hemosiderin granules without Prussian blue stain ($\times 500$).
57. CSF—macrophage with hemosiderin and hematoidin crystals: Notice yellow-orange color of crystals ($\times 500$).
58. CSF—malignant melanoma cell containing dustlike granules: Granules are much finer than hemosiderin granules ($\times 500$).
59. CSF—choroid plexus cells: Can be distinguished from malignant cells by the nuclear uniformity and distinct cell borders ($\times 500$).
60. CSF—ependymal cells ($\times 500$).
61. CSF—eosinophils: Notice cytocentrifuge distortion ($\times 1000$).
62. CSF—nucleated red blood cells seen with bone marrow contamination ($\times 500$).
63. CSF—broad spectrum of lymphocytes seen with viral meningitis ($\times 500$).
64. CSF—neutrophils with intracellular bacteria seen in bacterial meningitis ($\times 500$).
65. CSF—cryptococcus with budding form ($\times 250$).
66. CSF—lymphoblasts from acute lymphocytic leukemia: Observe prominent nucleoli ($\times 500$).
67. CSF—lymphoma cells: Notice prominent nucleoli and fine nuclear chromatin ($\times 500$).
68. CSF—Burkitt's lymphoma: Notice characteristic vacuoles ($\times 500$).
69. CSF—myeloblasts from acute myelocytic leukemia: Notice prominent nucleoli ($\times 500$).

70. CSF—monoblasts and two normal lymphocytes ($\times$ 1000).

71. CSF—normal mesothelial cell ($\times$ 500).

72. CSF—adenocarcinoma of prostate showing nuclear molding and hyperchromatic macronucleoli ($\times$ 500).

73. Seminal fluid: Normal spermatozoa ($\times$ 400).

74. Synovial fluid: Polarized uric acid crystals; intracellular needle-shaped crystals ($\times$ 500).

75. Synovial fluid: Polarized calcium pyrophosphate crystals; intracellular rhombic-shaped crystals ($\times$ 500).

76. Synovial fluid: Compensated polarized uric acid crystals; yellow crystal is aligned with the slow vibration ($\times$ 500).

77. Synovial fluid: Compensated polarized calcium pyrophosphate crystals; blue crystal is aligned with the slow vibration ($\times$ 500).

78. Pleural fluid: Plasma cells seen in tuberculosis ($\times$ 500).

79. Pleural fluid: Reactive mesothelial cells showing eccentric nuclei and vacuoles ($\times$ 500).

80. Pleural fluid: One normal and two reactive mesothelial cells with multinucleated form ($\times$ 250).

81. Pleural fluid: Adenocarcinoma showing nuclear molding ($\times$ 250).

82. Pleural fluid: Poorly differentiated adenocarcinoma showing nuclear irregularities ($\times$ 500).

83. Pleural fluid: Small cell carcinoma showing "Indian file" molding ($\times$ 250).

84. Pleural fluid: Nuclear enhancement as seen with toluidine-blue/horse serum stain showing nuclear irregularities ($\times$ 500).

85. Pericardial fluid: Adenocarcinoma showing nuclear irregularities ($\times$ 500).

86. Peritoneal fluid: Budding yeast ($\times$ 400).

87. Peritoneal fluid: Lipophages (macrophages containing fat) ($\times$ 500).

88. Peritoneal fluid: Ovarian carcinoma showing large mucin containing vacuoles ($\times$ 500).

89. Peritoneal fluid: Ovarian carcinoma showing community borders, nuclear irregularities, and hypochromatic macronucleoli ($\times$ 500).

90. Peritoneal fluid: Psammoma bodies showing concentric striation ($\times$ 500).

COLOR PLATES 1 THROUGH 90

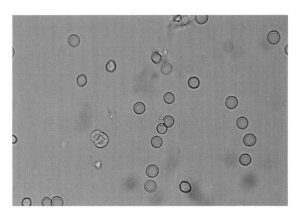

1. Normal red blood cells, one white blood cell (magnification ×400).

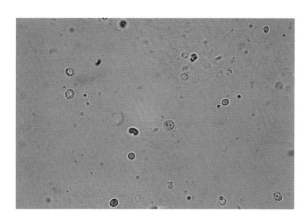

2. Red blood cells: crenated and dysmorphic forms (magnification ×400).

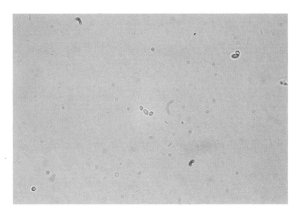

3. Yeast: Budding form aids in identification (magnification ×400).

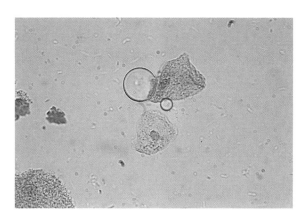

4. Oil droplets: Notice the refractility commonly found with artifacts (magnification ×400).

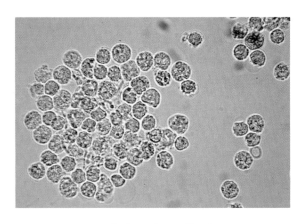

5. White blood cell clump (magnification ×400).

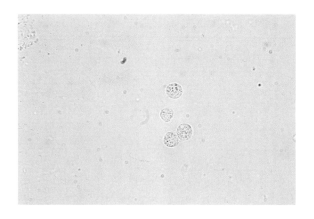

6. White blood cells (magnification ×400).

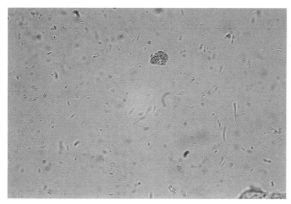

7. Stained white blood cells and bacteria (magnification × 400).

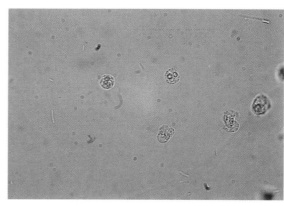

8. White blood cells with acetic acid: Nuclear detail is enhanced by 2 percent acetic acid (magnification × 400).

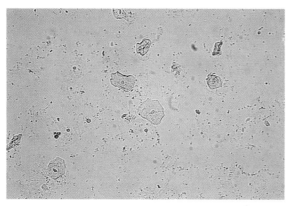

9. Squamous epithelial cells: Irregularly shaped, easily identified under low power (magnification × 100).

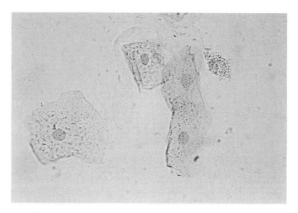

10. Stained squamous epithelial cells (magnification × 400).

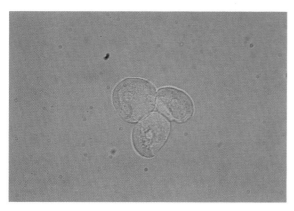

11. Transitional epithelial cells (magnification × 400).

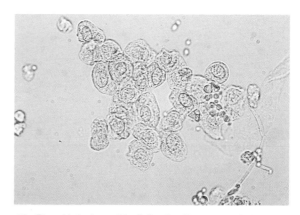

12. Renal tubular epithelial cells: Presence of single nucleus differentiates these from WBCs (magnification × 400).

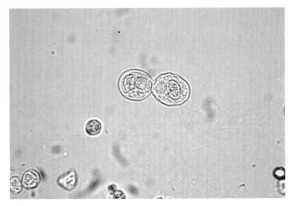

13. Renal tubular epithelial cells and white blood cells: Notice differences in size and nuclear structure (magnification ×400).

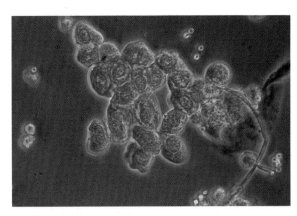

14. Renal tubular epithelial cells under phase (magnification ×400).

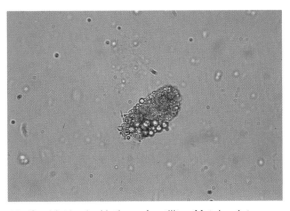

15. Oval fat body: Notice refractility of fat droplets (magnification ×400).

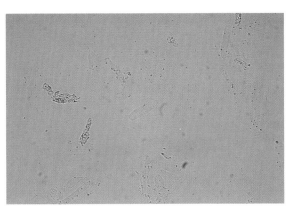

16. Hyaline casts and mucus: Low refractive index of both elements requires reduced light to prevent overlooking them. Compare the consistent form of the casts to the irregularly shaped mucus (magnification ×100).

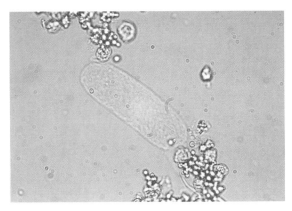

17. Hyaline cast (magnification ×400).

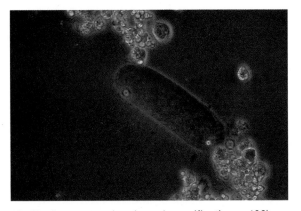

18. Hyaline cast under phase (magnification ×400).

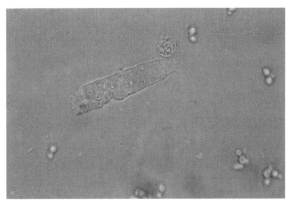

19. Convoluted hyaline cast: Notch suggests progression to waxy form (magnification × 400).

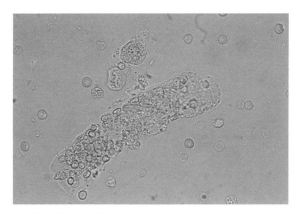

20. Red blood cell cast: Notice the presence of free red blood cells, including ghost cells (magnification × 400).

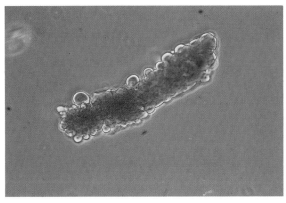

21. Stained red blood cell cast under phase (magnification × 400).

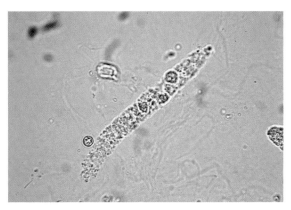

22. White blood cell and granular cast: Granules suggest white blood cell disintegration (magnification × 400).

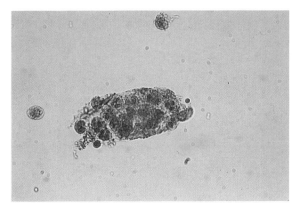

23. Stained white blood cell cast (magnification × 400).

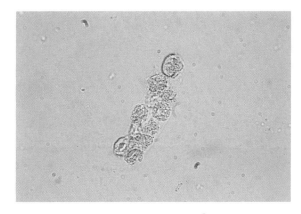

24. Renal tubular epithelial cell cast: Observe the surface attachment of cells to the cast matrix (magnification × 400).

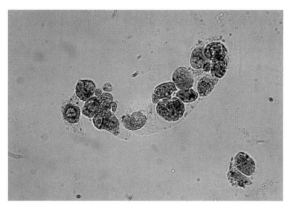

25. Stained renal tubular epithelial cell cast (magnification × 400).

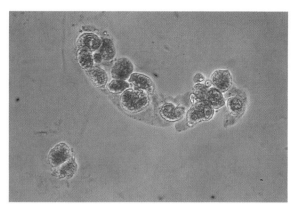

26. Stained renal tubular epithelial cell cast under phase (magnification × 400).

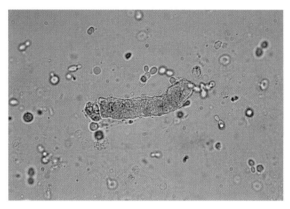

27. Coarsely granular cast with hemoglobin pigment: A comparison of red blood cells and yeast can also be made from this slide (magnification × 400).

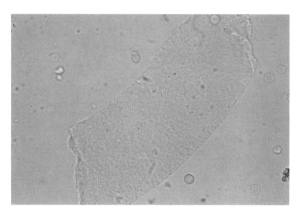

28. Waxy cast: Notice the irregularly broken ends (magnification × 400).

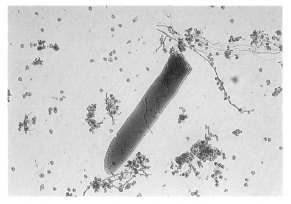

29. Stained waxy cast, white blood cells, and yeast (magnification × 100).

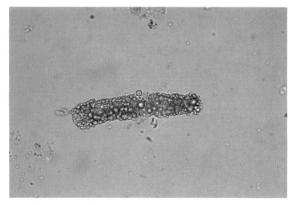

30. Fatty cast: Observe the refractile fat droplets on the matrix surface (magnification × 400).

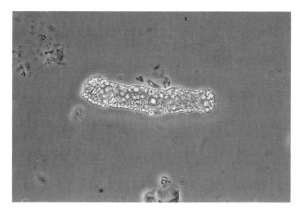

31. Fatty cast under phase (magnification ×400).

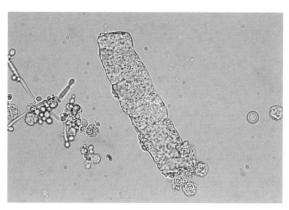

32. Broad granular cast (magnification ×400).

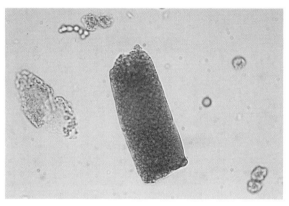

33. Stained broad granular cast (magnification ×400).

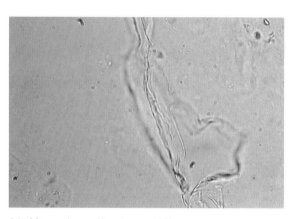

34. Mucus (magnification ×400).

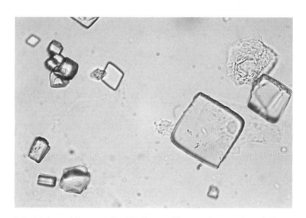

35. Uric acid crystals: Notice yellow color and variety of shapes (magnification ×400).

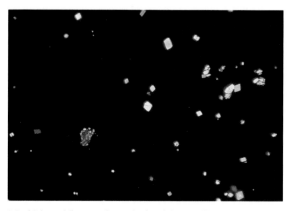

36. Uric acid crystals, polarized (magnification ×100).

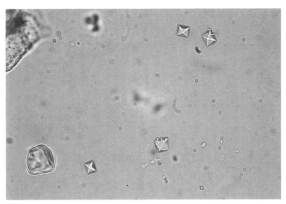

37. Calcium oxalate crystals: Notice classic "envelope" appearance (magnification × 400).

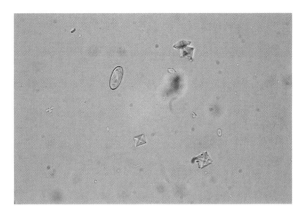

38. Oval and classic calcium oxalate crystals (magnification × 400).

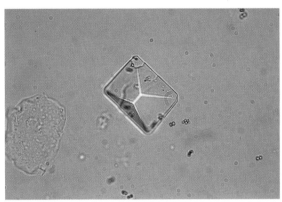

39. Triple phosphate crystals: Notice classic "coffin lid" appearance (magnification × 400).

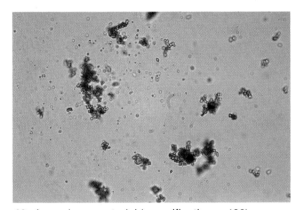

40. Amorphous material (magnification × 400).

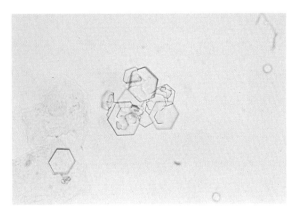

41. Cystine crystals: Notice colorless, hexagonal plates (magnification × 400).

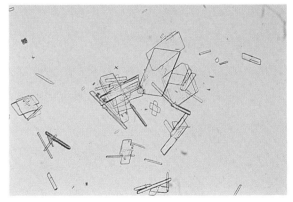

42. Cholesterol crystals: Notice notched corners on many plates (magnification × 100).

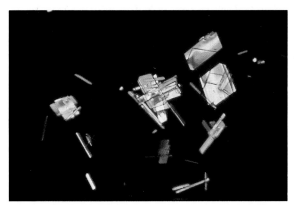

43. Cholesterol crystals, polarized (magnification × 100).

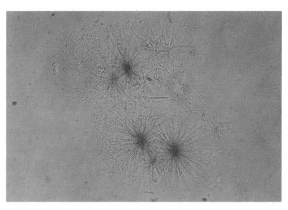

44. Tyrosine crystals: Yellow color suggests presence of liver disease (magnification × 400).

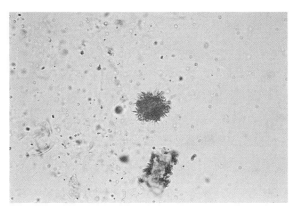

45. Bilirubin crystals: Observe the classic yellow color (magnification × 400).

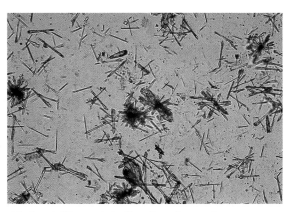

46. Ampicillin crystals: Bundles of crystals are seen following refrigeration (magnification × 100).

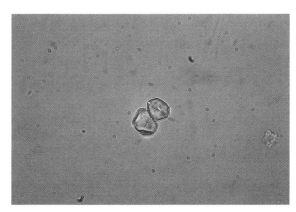

47. Starch granules: Notice refractility (magnification × 400).

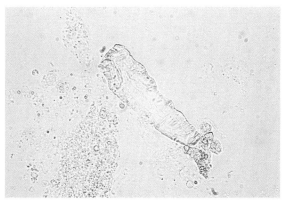

48. Artifact resembling waxy cast: Notice the lack of typical cast form and the refractility (magnification × 400).

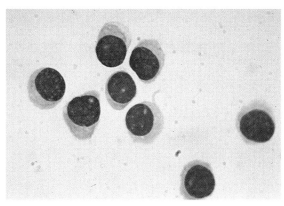

49. CSF—normal lymphocytes: Some cytocentrifuge distortion of cytoplasm (magnification × 1000).

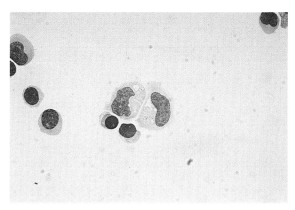

50. CSF—normal lymphocytes and monocytes (magnification × 500).

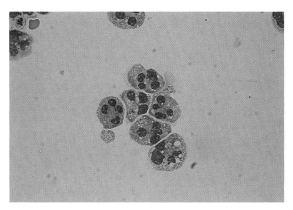

51. CSF—neutrophils: Cytoplasmic vacuoles result from cytocentrifugation (magnification × 500).

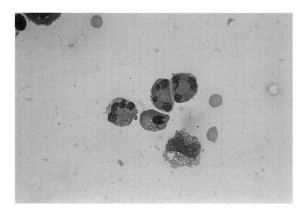

52. CSF—neutrophils with pyknotic nuclei (magnification × 500).

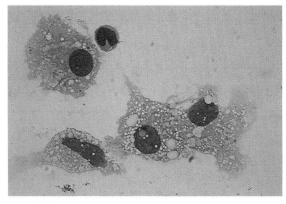

53. CSF—macrophages: Notice presence of large vacuoles (magnification × 500).

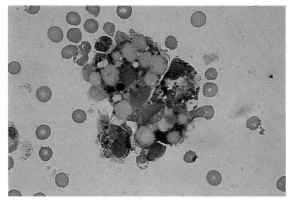

54. CSF—macrophages showing erythrophagocytosis (magnification × 500).

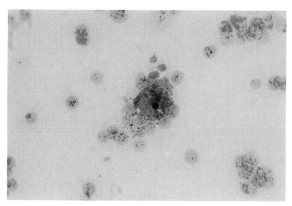

55. CSF—macrophage containing hemosiderin stained with Prussian blue (magnification × 25).

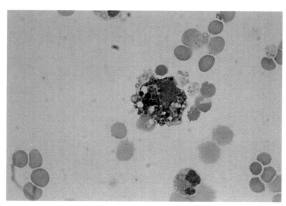

56. CSF—macrophage with large aggregated hemosiderin granules without Prussian blue stain (magnification × 500).

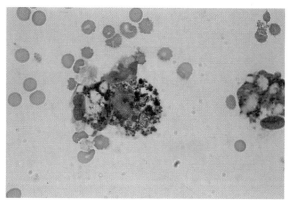

57. CSF—macrophage with hemosiderin and hematoidin crystals: Notice yellow-orange color of crystals (magnification × 500).

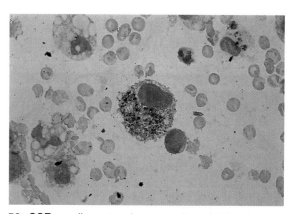

58. CSF—malignant melanoma cell containing dust-like granules: Granules are much finer than hemosiderin granules (magnification × 500).

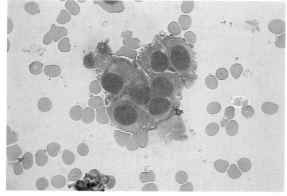

59. CSF—choroid plexus cells: Can be distinguished from malignant cells by the nuclear uniformity and distinct cell borders (magnification × 500).

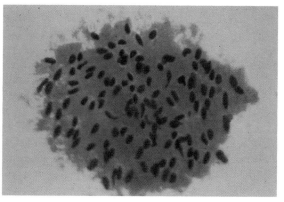

60. CSF—ependymal cells (magnification × 500).

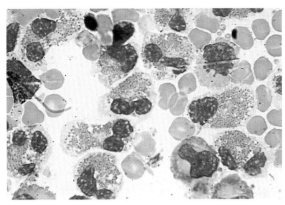

61. CSF—eosinophils: Notice cytocentrifuge distortion (magnification ×1000).

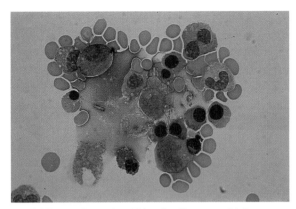

62. CSF—nucleated red blood cells seen with bone marrow contamination (magnification ×500).

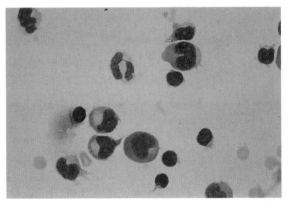

63. CSF—broad spectrum of lymphocytes seen with viral meningitis (magnification ×500).

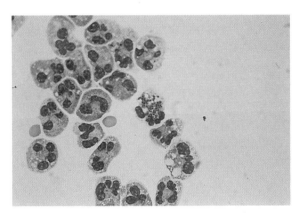

64. CSF—neutrophils with intracellular bacteria seen in bacterial meningitis (magnification ×500).

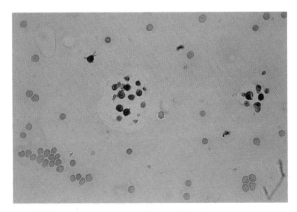

65. CSF—cryptococcus with budding form (magnification ×250).

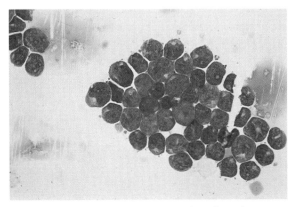

66. CSF—lymphoblasts from acute lymphocytic leukemia: Observe prominent nucleoli (magnification ×500).

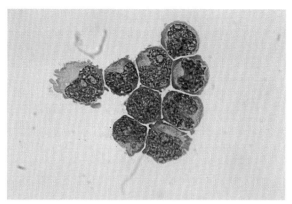

67. CSF—lymphoma cells: Notice prominent nucleoli and fine nuclear chromatin (magnification ×500).

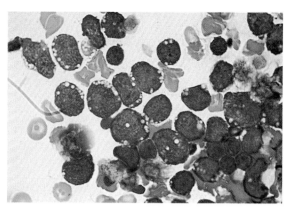

68. CSF—Burkitt's lymphoma: Notice characteristic vacuoles (magnification ×500).

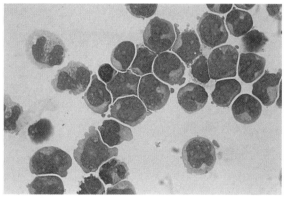

69. CSF—myeloblasts from acute myelocytic leukemia: Notice prominent nucleoli (magnification ×500).

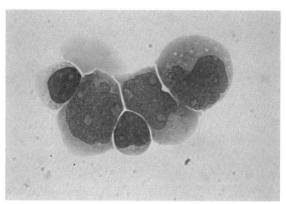

70. CSF—monoblasts and two normal lymphocytes (magnification ×1000).

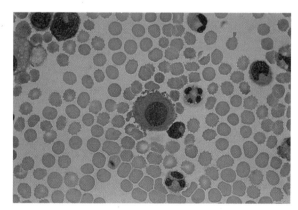

71. CSF—Normal mesothelial cell (magnification ×500).

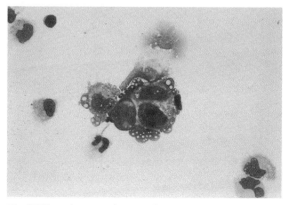

72. CSF—adenocarcinoma of prostate showing nuclear molding and hyperchromatic macronucleoli (magnification ×500).

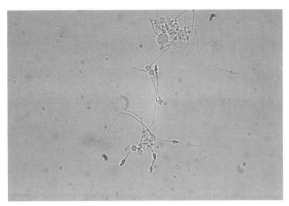

73. Seminal fluid: Normal spermatozoa (magnification ×400).

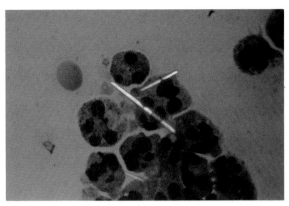

74. Synovial fluid: Polarized uric acid crystals; intracellular needle-shaped crystals (magnification ×500).

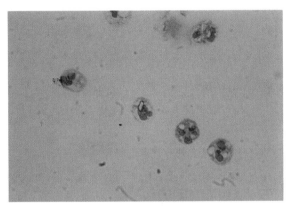

75. Synovial fluid: Polarized calcium pyrophosphate crystals; intracellular rhombic-shaped crystals (magnification ×500).

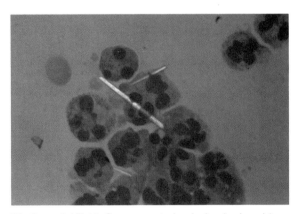

76. Synovial fluid: Compensated polarized uric acid crystals; yellow crystal is aligned with the slow vibration (magnification ×500).

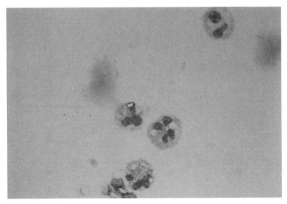

77. Synovial fluid: Compensated polarized calcium pyrophosphate crystals; blue crystal is aligned with the slow vibration (magnification ×500).

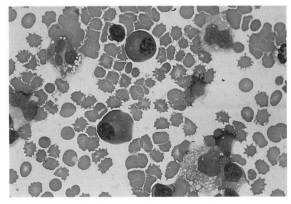

78. Pleural fluid: Plasma cells seen in tuberculosis (magnification ×500).

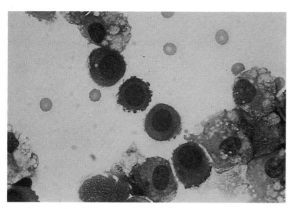

79. Pleural fluid: Reactive mesothelial cells showing eccentric nuclei and vacuoles (magnification ×500).

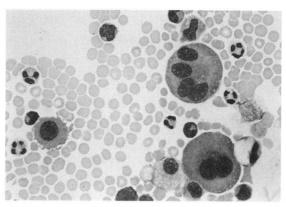

80. Pleural fluid: One normal and two reactive mesothelial cells with multinucleated form (magnification ×250).

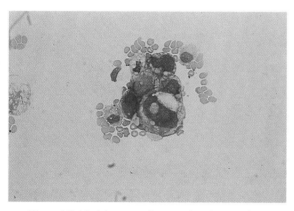

81. Pleural fluid: Adenocarcinoma showing nuclear molding (magnification ×250).

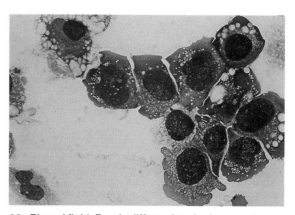

82. Pleural fluid: Poorly differentiated adenocarcinoma showing nuclear irregularities (magnification ×500).

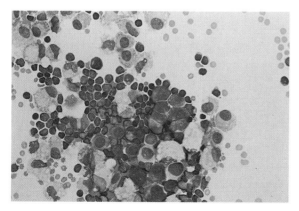

83. Pleural fluid: Small cell carcinoma showing "Indian file" molding (magnification ×250).

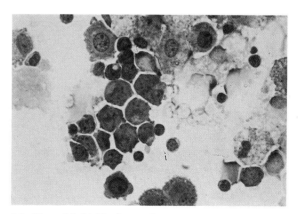

84. Pleural fluid: Nuclear enhancement as seen with toluidine-blue/horse serum stain showing nuclear irregularities (magnification ×500).

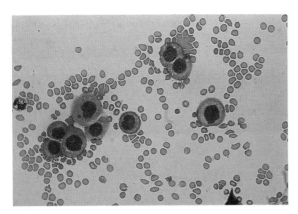

85. Pericardial fluid: Adenocarcinoma showing nuclear irregularities (magnification ×500).

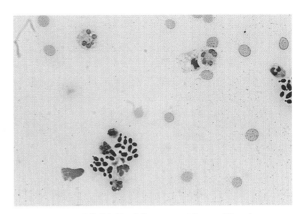

86. Peritoneal fluid: Budding yeast (magnification ×400).

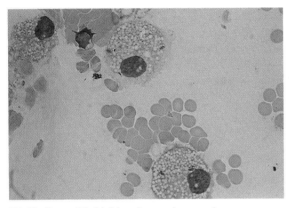

87. Peritoneal fluid: Lipophages (macrophages containing fat) (magnification ×500).

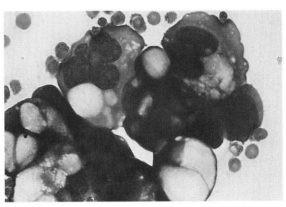

88. Peritoneal fluid: Ovarian carcinoma showing large mucin containing vacuoles (magnification ×500).

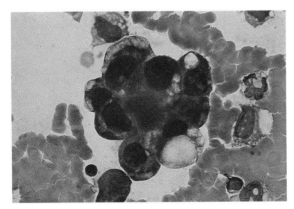

89. Peritoneal fluid: Ovarian carcinoma showing community borders, nuclear irregularities, and hypochromatic macronucleoli (magnification ×500).

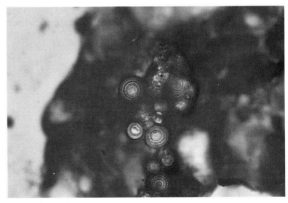

90. Peritoneal fluid: Psammoma bodies showing concentric striation (magnification ×500).

1

INTRODUCTION TO URINALYSIS

LEARNING OBJECTIVES

Upon completion of this chapter, readers will be able to

1. list three major chemical constituents of urine.
2. describe a method for determining whether a questionable fluid is urine.
3. list three basic rules for specimen handling and explain their importance.
4. recognize normal and abnormal daily urine volumes.
5. briefly discuss five methods for preserving urine specimens, including their advantages and disadvantages.
6. list eight changes that may take place in a urine specimen that remains at room temperature for more than 2 hours.
7. instruct a patient in the correct procedure for collecting a timed urine specimen.
8. describe the type of specimen needed to obtain optimal results when a specific urinalysis procedure is requested.
9. define the common terms encountered in urinalysis and use them in proper context.
10. recognize common abbreviations associated with urinalysis and tell what they represent.

HISTORY AND IMPORTANCE

The analysis of urine was actually the beginning of laboratory medicine. References to the study of urine can be found in the drawings of the cavemen and in Egyptian hieroglyphics such as the Edwin Smith Surgical Papyrus. Pictures of early physicians, called "pisse prophets," commonly showed them examining a glass or flask of urine. Often, these physicians never saw the patient, only the patient's urine. Although these physicians lacked the sophisticated testing mechanisms now available, they were able to obtain diagnostic information from such basic observations as color, turbidity, odor, volume, viscosity, and even sweetness, inasmuch as certain specimens attracted ants. It is interesting to note that these same urine characteristics are still reported by laboratory personnel today. However, modern urinalysis has expanded its scope to include not only the physical examination of urine but also the chemical analysis and microscopic examination of the urinary sediment.

Many well-known names in the history of medicine are associated with the study of urine, including Hippocrates, who in the fifth century BC wrote a book on "uroscopy."

Physicians concentrated their efforts very heavily on the art of "uroscopy." By 1140 AD, color charts had been developed that described the significance of 20 different colors. Chemical testing progressed from "ant testing" and "taste testing" for glucose to Frederik Dekkers'discovery, in 1694, of albuminuria by boiling urine and on to the measurement of urinary gold, silver, and lead in the 1800s.[5] The invention of the microscope in the 17th century led to the examination of urinary sediment and to the development by Thomas Addis of methods for quantitating the microscopic sediment. Urinalysis was introduced as part of a doctor's routine patient examination by Richard Bright in 1827. However, by the 1930s, the number and complexity of the tests performed in a urinalysis had reached a point of impracticality, and the urinalysis began to disappear from routine examinations. Fortunately, the development of modern testing techniques rescued the routine urinalysis, and it has remained an integral part of the patient examination.

Two unique characteristics of a urine specimen can account for this continued popularity:

1. Urine is a readily available and easily collected specimen.
2. Urine contains information about many of the body's major metabolic functions, and this information can be obtained by simple laboratory tests.

These characteristics fit in well with the current trends toward preventive medicine and lower medical costs. By offering an inexpensive way to test large numbers of people not only for renal disease but also for the asymptomatic beginnings of conditions such as diabetes mellitus and liver disease, the urinalysis can be a very valuable metabolic screening procedure. However, care must be taken in the laboratory not to let the simplicity of the procedure result in a relaxation of testing standards, and care must be taken by physicians to order the test in a cost-effective manner.[6]

FORMATION

Urine is continuously formed by the kidneys. It is actually an ultrafiltrate of plasma from which glucose, amino acids, water, and other substances essential to body metabolism have been reabsorbed. The physiologic process by which approximately 170,000 ml of filtered plasma is converted to the average daily urine output of 1200 ml is discussed in detail in chapter 2.

COMPOSITION

In general, urine consists of urea and other organic and inorganic chemicals dissolved in water. Considerable variations in the concentrations of these substances can occur due to the influence of factors such as dietary intake, physical activity, body metabolism, endocrine function, and even body position. Urea, a metabolic waste product produced in the liver from the breakdown of protein and amino acids, accounts for nearly half of the total dissolved solids in urine. Other organic substances include primarily creatinine and uric acid. The major inorganic solid dissolved in urine is chloride, followed by sodium and potassium. Small or trace amounts of many additional inorganic chemicals are also present in urine. The concentrations of these inorganic compounds are greatly influenced by dietary intake, making it difficult to establish normal levels. Table 1–1 shows the major chemical substances in urine. Other substances found in urine include hormones, vitamins, and medications. Although not a part of the original plasma filtrate, the urine may also contain formed elements such as cells, crystals, mucus, and bacteria. Increased amounts of these formed elements are often indicative of disease. Should it be necessary to determine whether a particular fluid is actually urine, the specimen can be tested for its urea and creatinine content. Inasmuch as both of these substances are present in much higher concentrations in urine than in other body fluids, the demonstration of a high urea and creatinine content can identify a fluid as urine.[2]

TABLE 1–1. Composition of Urine*

COMPONENT	AMOUNT		URINE/PLASMA RATIO
Sodium	2–4 g	100–200 mEq	0.8–1.5
Potassium	1.5–2.0 g	50–70 mEq	10–15
Magnesium	0.1–0.2 g	8–16 mEq	
Calcium	0.1–0.3 g	2.5–7.5 mEq	
Iron	0.2 mg		
Ammonia	0.4–1.0 g N	30–75 mEq	
H^+		$4 \times 10^{-8} - 4 \times 10^{-6}$ mEq/liter	1–100
Uric acid	0.80–0.2 g N		20
Amino acids	0.08–0.15 g N		
Hippuric acid	0.04–0.08 g N		
Chloride		100–250 mEq	0.8–2
Bicarbonate		0–50 mEq	0–2
Phosphate	0.7–1.6 g P	20–50 mmol	25
Inorganic sulfate	0.6–1.8 g S	40–120 mEq	50
Organic sulfate	0.06–0.2 g S		
Urea	6–18 g N		35
Creatinine	0.3–0.8 g N		70
Peptides	0.3–0.7 g N		

*The values indicate the average contents of adult human urine collected for 24 hours.
(From White, A, et al: Principles of Biochemistry, ed 6. McGraw-Hill, New York, 1978, p 1076, with permission.)

VOLUME

Urine volume is dependent upon the amount of water excreted by the kidneys. Water is a major body constituent; therefore, the amount excreted is usually determined by the body's state of hydration. Factors that influence urine volume include fluid intake; fluid loss from nonrenal sources; variations in the secretion of antidiuretic hormone; and the necessity to excrete increased amounts of dissolved solids, such as glucose or salts. Taking these factors into consideration, it can be seen that although the average daily urine output is 1200 to 1500 ml, a range of 600 to 2000 ml may be considered normal.[2]

Oliguria, a decrease in the normal daily urine volume, is commonly seen when the body enters a state of dehydration due to excessive water loss from vomiting, diarrhea, perspiration, or severe burns. Oliguria leading to anuria, cessation of urine flow, may result from any serious damage to the kidneys or from a decrease in the flow of blood to the kidneys. Two or three times more urine is excreted during the day than during the night. An increase in the nocturnal excretion of urine is termed nocturia. Polyuria, an increase in daily urine volume, is often associated with diabetes mellitus and diabetes insipidus; however, it may also be artificially induced by the use of diuretics, caffeine, or alcohol, all of which suppress the secretion of antidiuretic hormone.

Diabetes mellitus and diabetes insipidus produce polyuria for different reasons, and analysis of the urine is an important step in the differential diagnosis. Diabetes mellitus is caused by a defect either in the production of insulin by the pancreas or in the function of insulin, resulting in an increased body glucose concentration. The excess glucose is not reabsorbed by the kidneys, necessitating the excretion of increased amounts of water to remove the dissolved glucose from the body. Although appearing to be dilute, a urine specimen from a patient with diabetes mellitus will have a high specific gravity because of the increased glucose content. Diabetes insipidus results from a decrease in the production or function of antidiuretic hormone; thus, the water necessary for adequate body hydration is not reabsorbed from the plasma filtrate. In this condition, the urine will be truly dilute and will have a low specific gravity. Fluid loss in both diseases is compensated for by increased ingestion of water, producing an even greater urine volume. Polyuria accompanied by increased fluid intake is often the first symptom of either disease.

SPECIMEN COLLECTION

The fact that a urine specimen is so readily available and easily collected often leads to laxity in the treatment of the specimen after it has been collected. Changes in urine composition take place not only in vivo but also in vitro, thus necessitating correct handling procedures after the specimen is collected.

Three major rules of urine specimen handling actually apply to all specimens received in the laboratory:

1. The specimen must be collected in a clean, dry container. Disposable containers are becoming increasingly more popular because they are cost effective and the chance of contamination owing to improper washing is eliminated. These disposable containers are available in a variety of sizes and shapes, including plastic bags with adhesive for the collection of pediatric specimens and large containers for 24-hour specimens.
2. The specimen containers must be properly labeled with the patient's name, the date and time of collection, and, when appropriate, additional information such as the hospital number and the doctor's name. Remember, several unlabeled urine specimens sitting on their respective requisition slips can easily be moved.
3. The specimen must be delivered to the laboratory promptly and tested within 1 hour. A specimen that cannot be delivered or tested within 1 hour should be refrigerated or have an appropriate chemical preservative added.

PRESERVATION

The most routinely used method of preservation is refrigeration, which is reliable in preventing bacterial decomposition of urine for an overnight period.[14] Refrigeration of the specimen can cause an increase in the specific gravity and the precipitation of amorphous phosphates and urates which may obscure the microscopic sediment analysis. However, allowing the specimen to return to room temperature prior to analysis will correct the specific gravity and may dissolve some of the amorphous urates. When a specimen must be transported over a long distance and refrigeration is not possible, chemical preservatives may be added. The ideal preservative should be bactericidal, inhibit urease, and preserve formed elements in the sediment. At the same time, it should not interfere with chemical tests.[3] Unfortunately, as can be seen in Table 1–2, the ideal preservative does not presently exist; therefore, it is important to choose a preservative that best suits the needs of the required analysis.

CHANGES IN UNPRESERVED URINE

Problems introduced by preservation can be considered minor if one considers the changes that take place in unpreserved urine. The following 10 changes may occur in a specimen allowed to remain unpreserved at room temperature for longer than 1 hour:

1. increased **pH** from the breakdown of urea to ammonia by urease-producing bacteria
2. decreased **glucose** due to glycolysis and bacterial utilization
3. decreased **ketones** because of volatilization
4. decreased **bilirubin** from exposure to light
5. decreased **urobilinogen** by its oxidation to urobilin
6. increased **nitrite** due to bacterial reduction of nitrate

7. increased **bacteria**
8. increased **turbidity** caused by bacterial growth and possible precipitation of amorphous material
9. disintegration of **red blood cells** and **casts,** particularly in dilute alkaline urine
10. changes in **color** due to oxidation or reduction of metabolites.

These variations will be discussed again under the individual test procedures. At this point, it is important to realize that the results of a routine urinalysis can be seriously affected by improper preservation.

TABLE 1–2. Urine Preservatives

PRESERVATIVE	ADVANTAGES	DISADVANTAGES	ADDITIONAL INFORMATION
Refrigeration	No interference with chemical tests	Raises specific gravity by hydrometer Precipitates amorphous phosphates and urates	Shown to prevent bacterial growth for at least 24 hours[14]
Thymol	Preserves glucose and sediments well	Interferes with acid precipitation tests for protein Large amounts will interfere with o-toluidine glucose tests	
Boric acid	Preserves protein and formed elements well[11] No interference with routine analyses other than pH	Large amounts are needed to inhibit bacterial growth Large amounts may cause crystal precipitation	Keeps pH at about 6.0 Interferes with drug and hormone analyses[9]
Formalin (formaldehyde)	Excellent sediment preservative	Interferes with copper reduction tests for glucose Causes clumping of sediment[11]	Containers for collection of specimens for cell counts can be rinsed with formalin for better preservation of cells and casts
Chloroform	None	Sinks to the bottom of the specimen and interferes with sediment analysis Interferes with "falling drop" specific gravity	May cause cellular changes

(continued)

Table 1–2. *Continued*

PRESERVATIVE	ADVANTAGES	DISADVANTAGES	ADDITIONAL INFORMATION
Toluene	Does not interfere with routine chemical tests	Floats on the surface of specimens and clings to pipettes and testing materials	
Sodium fluoride	Prevents glycolysis Good preservative for drug analyses[9]	Inhibits dipstick tests for glucose	Will not interfere with hexokinase tests for glucose Sodium benzoate instead of fluoride may be used for dipstick testing[8]
Hydrochloric acid	Bactericidal	Destroys formed elements and precipitates solutes Unacceptable for routine analysis	May be dangerous to the patient[3]
Freezing	Preserves bilirubin and urobilinogen	Destroys formed elements Turbidity occurs upon thawing	Useful for nonroutine chemical analyses[7]
Commercial preservative tablets	Convenient when refrigeration is not possible Chemical concentration is controlled to minimize interference	May increase specific gravity[5] May contain one or more of the above chemical preservatives	Check tablet composition to determine possible effects on desired tests
Urine C + S Transport Kit (Becton Dickinson, Rutherford, NJ 07070)	Urinalysis and culture can be run on same specimen	Increases specific gravity and protein Decreases pH	Not as cost effective as refrigeration

TYPES OF SPECIMENS

To obtain a specimen that is truly representative of a patient's metabolic state, it is often necessary to regulate certain aspects of specimen collection. These special conditions may include time of collection, length of collection, patient's dietary and medicinal in-

TABLE 1–3. Types of Urine Specimens

TYPE OF SPECIMEN	PURPOSE
Random	Routine screening
First morning	Routine screening Pregnancy tests Orthostatic protein
Fasting	Diabetic monitoring
2-Hour postprandial	Diabetic monitoring Glucose testing
Glucose tolerance test (GTT)	Accompanies blood samples in glucose tolerance test
24-hour (or timed)	Quantitative chemical tests
Catheterized	Bacterial culture
Midstream clean-catch	Routine screening Bacterial culture
Suprapubic aspiration	Bladder urine for bacterial culture Cytology

take, and method of collection. It is important to instruct patients when special collection procedures must be followed. Frequently encountered specimens are listed in Table 1–3.

RANDOM SPECIMEN

This is the most commonly received specimen due to the ease of collection and the lack of inconvenience to the patient. The random specimen is useful for routine screening tests to detect obvious abnormalities. However, it may also produce erroneous results caused by dietary intake or physical activity just prior to the collection of the specimen. The patient will then be requested to collect additional specimens under more controlled conditions.

FIRST MORNING SPECIMEN

Although it may require the patient to make an additional trip to the laboratory, this is the ideal screening specimen. It is also essential for preventing false-negative pregnancy tests and for evaluating orthostatic proteinuria. The first morning specimen is a concentrated specimen, thereby assuring detection of substances that may not be present in a dilute random specimen. The patient should be instructed to collect the specimen immediately upon arising and to deliver it to the laboratory within 2 hours.

FASTING SPECIMEN

A fasting specimen differs from a first morning specimen by being the second voided specimen after a period of fasting. This specimen will not contain any metabolites from food ingested prior to the beginning of the fasting period and is recommended for glucose monitoring.[4]

2-Hour Postprandial Specimen

The patient is instructed to void shortly before consuming a routine meal and to collect a specimen 2 hours after eating. The specimen is tested for glucose, and the results are used primarily for monitoring insulin therapy in persons with diabetes mellitus. A more comprehensive evaluation of the patient's status can be obtained if the results of the 2-hour postprandial specimen are compared with those of a fasting specimen.

Glucose Tolerance Test (GTT) Specimens

These specimens are collected to correspond with the blood samples drawn during a glucose tolerance test. The number of specimens varies with the length of the test. All tests will include fasting, ½-hour, 1-hour, 2-hour, and 3-hour specimens, and possibly 4-, 5-, and 6-hour specimens. The urine is tested for glucose and ketones, and the results are reported with the blood test results as an aid to interpreting the patient's ability to metabolize a measured amount of glucose.

24-Hour (or Timed) Specimen

Often, it is necessary to measure the exact amount of a urine chemical rather than to report just its presence or absence. A carefully timed specimen must be used to produce accurate quantitative results. When the concentration of the substance to be measured varies with daily activities such as exercise, meals, and body metabolism, a 24-hour collection is required. If the concentration of the particular substance remains constant, the specimen may be collected over a shorter period of time. However, care must be taken to keep the patient adequately hydrated during short collection periods. Patients must be explicitly instructed on the procedure for collecting a timed specimen. To obtain an accurately timed specimen, it is necessary to begin the collection period with an empty bladder and to end the collection period with an empty bladder. The following instructions for collecting a 24-hour specimen can be applied to any timed collection.

Day 1–7 AM: Patient voids and **discards** specimen. Patient **collects** all urine for the next 24 hours.
Day 2–7 AM: Patient voids and **adds** this urine to the previously collected urine.

Upon its arrival in the laboratory, a 24-hour specimen must be thoroughly mixed and the volume accurately measured and recorded. If only an aliquot is needed for testing, the amount saved must be adequate to permit repeat or additional testing, if necessary. Consideration must also be given to the preservation of specimens collected over extended periods of time. The preservative chosen should be nontoxic to the patient and should not interfere with the tests to be performed. Appropriate collection information is included with test procedures and should be referred to before issuing a container and instructions to the patient. To ensure the accuracy of a 24-hour specimen, a known quantity of a nontoxic chemical marker, such as 4-aminobenzoic acid, may be given to the patient at the start of the collection period. The concentration of excreted marker in the specimen is measured to determine the completeness of the collection. Use of an injected inert marker the concentration of which can be controlled is recommended over measurement of endogenous urine creatinine, which varies with dietary intake and body mass.[1]

Catheterized Specimen

This specimen is collected under sterile conditions by passing a hollow tube through the urethra into the bladder. The most commonly requested test on a catheterized specimen is a bacterial culture. If a routine urinalysis is also requested, the culture should be performed first to prevent contamination of the specimen.

A less frequently encountered type of catheterized specimen is used to measure functions in the individual kidneys. Specimens from the right and left kidneys are collected separately by passing catheters through the ureters of the respective kidneys.

MIDSTREAM CLEAN-CATCH SPECIMEN

As an alternative to the catheterized specimen, the midstream clean-catch specimen provides a safer, less traumatic method for obtaining urine for bacterial culture. This specimen also offers a more representative and less contaminated specimen for microscopic analysis than the routinely voided specimen. Patients must be provided with appropriate cleansing materials and a sterile container. They must also be thoroughly instructed in the methods for cleansing the genitalia and for collecting only the midstream portion of the urine.

SUPRAPUBIC ASPIRATION

Occasionally, urine may be collected by external introduction of a needle into the bladder. Because the bladder is sterile under normal conditions, this collection method provides a sample for bacterial culture that is completely free of extraneous contamination. The specimen also can be used for cytologic examination.

PEDIATRIC SPECIMENS

Collection of pediatric specimens can present a challenge. Soft, clear plastic bags with adhesive to attach to the genital area of both boys and girls are available for collecting routine specimens. Sterile specimens are obtained by catheterization or by suprapubic aspiration. Quantitative chemical analysis can be performed on infant urine by extracting the urine from disposable diapers over a specified period of time.[12]

GLOSSARY

anuria. Complete stoppage of urine flow.
azotemia. Presence of increased nitrogenous waste products (primarily urea) in the blood.
catheter. Hollow tube for draining urine from the bladder or kidneys.
cystoscope. Instrument for examining the interior of the bladder and ureter.
diuresis. Passage of abnormally large amounts of urine.
diuretic. An agent that increases the formation of urine.
dysuria. Painful urination.
edema. Swelling due to excessive tissue fluid.
-emia. Relating to blood.
glycosuria (glucosuria). Glucose in the urine.
hematuria. Blood in the urine.
hypersthenuria. Urine with a specific gravity greater than the 1.010 specific gravity of the plasma filtrate.
hyposthenuria. Urine with a specific gravity less than the 1.010 specific gravity of the plasma filtrate.
isosthenuria. Urine with a specific gravity equal to the 1.010 specific gravity of the plasma filtrate.
ketonuria. Ketones in the urine.
nephritis. Inflammation of the kidney involving glomeruli, tubules, or interstitial tissue.
nephrology. The study of the structure and function of the kidney.
nocturia. Excessive urination during the night.
oliguria. Marked decrease in urine flow.
polydipsia. Excessive thirst.
polyuria. Marked increase in urine flow.

proteinuria (albuminuria). Protein in the urine.

pyuria. Pus in the urine.

refractometer. Instrument used for indirectly determining specific gravity by refractive index.

renal. Pertaining to the kidney.

renal calculi. Kidney stones.

renal dialysis. Procedure used to remove waste products from the blood when kidneys are not functioning.

uremia. Presence of increased urea in the blood.

-uria. Relating to the urine.

urinalysis (complete or routine). The physical, chemical, and microscopic analysis of urine.

urinometer (hydrometer). Instrument used for directly measuring the specific gravity of urine.

urologist. Physician specializing in the study of urology.

urology. Branch of medicine concerned with the male and female urinary tracts and the male genital tract.

ABBREVIATIONS

Abbreviation	Definition
ADH	Antidiuretic hormone
BJP	Bence Jones protein
BUN	Blood urea nitrogen
GTT	Glucose tolerance test
GU	Genitourinary
HCG	Human chorionic gonadotropin (pregnancy testing)
hpf	High-power field
IVP	Intravenous pyelogram (procedure performed in radiology using an opaque dye)
lpf	Low-power field
PKU	Phenylketonuria
2 hr pp or pc	Two hours after eating (postprandial or postcibal)
PSP	Phenolsulfonphthalein (dye used in renal function testing)
Q.C. or Q.A.	Quality control or assurance
qns	Quantity nonsufficient
RBC	red blood cell
Sp. Gr. or SG	Specific gravity
TNTC	Too numerous to count (e.g., WBC/hpf = TNTC)
UA	Routine urinalysis
WBC	White blood cell
WBC/hpf	Number of white blood cells seen per high-power field

REFERENCES

1. Bingham, S and Cummings, JH: The use of 4-aminobenzoic acid as a marker to validate the completeness of 24 hour urine collections in man. Clin Sci 64(6):629–635, 1984.
2. Bradley, B and Schumann, GB: Examination of urine. In Henry, JB (ed): Clinical Diagnosis and Management by Laboratory Methods. WB Saunders, Philadelphia, 1979.
3. Griffith, DP and Dunn, D: Collection and preservation of urine for biochemical analysis. Invest Urol 15(6):459–461, 1978.

4. Guthrie, D, Hinnen, D, and Guthrie, R: Single-voided vs. double-voided urine testing. Diabetes Care 2(3):269–271, 1979.

5. Herman, JR: Urology: A View Through the Retrospectroscope. Harper & Row, Hagerstown, Maryland, 1973.

6. Kiel, DP and Moskowitz, MA: The Urinalysis: A Critical Appraisal. Med Clin North Am 71(4):607–624, 1987.

7. Leach, CS, Rambault, PC, and Fischer, CL: A comparative study of two methods of urine preservation. Clin Biochem 8(2):108–117, 1975.

8. Onstad, J, Hancock, D, and Wolf, P: Inhibitory effect of fluoride on glucose tests with glucose oxidase strips. Clin Chem 21:898–899, 1975.

9. Porter, IA and Brodie, J: Boric acid preservation of urine samples. Br Med J 2:353–355, 1969.

10. Reilly, PA and Wians, FH: Evaluation of a urine transport kit on urine reagent strips. Lab Med 18(3):167–169, 1987.

11. Riddhimat, R, Tantiniti, P and Nilahul, C: Boric acid preservation of urine. Med Assoc Thai 68(9):473–479, 1985.

12. Roberts, SB and Lucas, A: Measurement of urinary constituents and output using disposable napkins. Arch Dis Child 60:1021–1024, 1985.

13. Rockerbie, RA and Campbell, DJ: Effect of specimen storage and preservation on toxicological analysis of urine. Clin Biochem 11(3):77–81, 1978.

14. Ryan, WL and Mills, RD: Bacterial multiplication in urine during refrigeration. Am J Med Technol 29:175–177, 1963.

STUDY QUESTIONS (Choose one best answer)

1. The primary chemical constituents of normal urine are

   a. water, protein, and sodium
   b. water, urea, and protein
   c. water, urea, and chloride
   d. water, urea, and bilirubin

2. A person exhibiting oliguria would have a daily urine volume of

   a. 200–600 ml
   b. 600–1000 ml
   c. 1000–1500 ml
   d. over 1500 ml

3. It is sometimes necessary to determine whether a specimen is actually urine. To do this, you would measure the concentration of

   a. glucose and ketones
   b. urea and creatinine
   c. uric acid and amino acids
   d. protein and amino acids

4. Urine from patients with diabetes mellitus has

   a. decreased volume and decreased specific gravity
   b. decreased volume and increased specific gravity
   c. increased volume and decreased specific gravity
   d. increased volume and increased specific gravity

5. A specimen containing precipitated amorphous phosphates may have been preserved using

   a. boric acid
   b. chloroform
   c. formalin
   d. refrigeration

6. For the best preservation of urinary sediments, the preservatives of choice are

   a. boric and hydrochloric acids
   b. formalin and boric acid
   c. formalin and freezing
   d. chloroform and refrigeration

7. An unpreserved specimen collected at 8 AM and remaining at room temperature until the afternoon shift arrives can be expected to have

   1 decreased glucose and ketones
   2 increased bacteria and nitrite
   3 decreased pH and turbidity
   4 decreased cellular elements

   a. 1, 2, and 3
   b. 1, 2, and 4
   c. 1 and 2 only
   d. 4 only

8. Red blood cells will disintegrate more rapidly in urine that is

   a. concentrated and acidic
   b. concentrated and alkaline
   c. dilute and acidic
   d. dilute and alkaline

9. Quantitative urine tests are most accurately performed on

   a. first morning specimens
   b. timed specimens
   c. midstream clean-catch specimens
   d. suprapubic aspirations

10. A first morning urine is the specimen of choice for routine urinalysis because

    a. it has a high volume
    b. it is produced while the body is in a resting state
    c. it is more concentrated, resulting in better detection of abnormalities
    d. it is more dilute, preventing false-positive reactions

11. Cessation of urine flow is termed

    a. azotemia
    b. dysuria
    c. diuresis
    d. anuria

12. Persons taking diuretics can be expected to produce

    a. proteinuria
    b. polyuria
    c. pyuria
    d. oliguria

13. Mary Johnson brings a urine specimen to the laboratory with a requisition for a glucose determination. The test is negative. Mary's doctor questions this result because she has a family history of diabetes mellitus and is experiencing mild clinical symptoms of the disease. What two possibilities regarding the urine specimen could account for a possible false-negative reaction with Mary's glucose test?

14. How could a specimen be obtained that would more accurately reflect Mary's glucose metabolism?

2

FUNCTION AND DISEASES OF THE KIDNEY

LEARNING OBJECTIVES

Upon completion of this chapter, readers will be able to

1. discuss the physiologic mechanisms of glomerular filtration, tubular reabsorption, tubular secretion, and renal blood flow.
2. identify the laboratory procedures used to evaluate these four renal functions.
3. differentiate between exogenous and endogenous procedures.
4. discuss the advantages and disadvantages in using urea, inulin, creatinine, β_2 microglobulin, and radionucleotides for the measurement of glomerular filtration.
5. given hypothetic laboratory data, calculate a creatinine clearance and determine if the result is normal.
6. describe the Fishberg and Mosenthal concentration tests, including specimen collection, testing, and normal results.
7. define osmolarity and discuss its relationship to urine concentration.
8. describe the basic principles of clinical osmometers.
9. given hypothetic laboratory data, calculate a free-water clearance and interpret the result.
10. discuss the principle and significance of the PSP test.
11. given hypothetic laboratory data, calculate a PAH clearance and relate this result to renal blood flow.
12. describe the relationship of urinary ammonia and titratable acidity to the production of an acidic urine.
13. state the primary cause of acute glomerulonephritis and describe the major urinalysis findings.
14. briefly discuss the chronic forms of glomerular disease, the nephrotic syndrome, and renal failure, including the renal functions affected and significant urinalysis results.
15. describe the urine sediment in pyelonephritis.

This chapter presents a review of nephron anatomy and physiology and its relationship to urinalysis and renal function testing, followed by a section on laboratory assessment of renal function and a discussion of the major renal diseases.

RENAL PHYSIOLOGY

Each kidney contains approximately 1 to 1.5 million nephrons. Figure 2–1 shows the relationship of the nephron to the kidney and excretory system, and Figure 2–2 provides

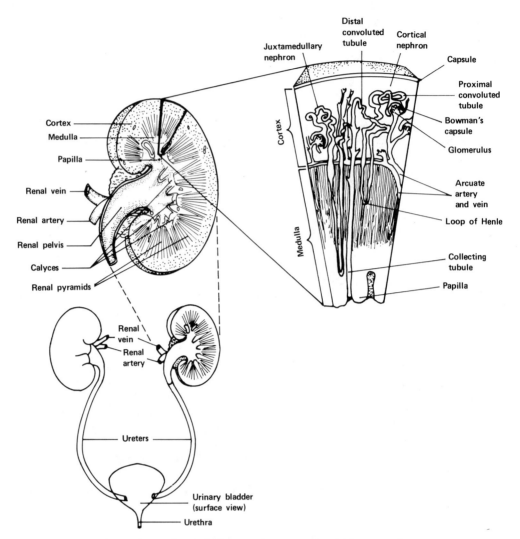

FIGURE 2–1. The relationship of the nephron to the kidney and excretory system. (Adapted from Spence, A and Mason, E: *Human Anatomy and Physiology.* Benjamin/ Cummings Publishing, Menlo Park, CA, 1987; and from Previte, J.J.: Human Physiology. McGraw-Hill, New York, 1983.)

a composite view of the nephron. The kidneys' ability to selectively clear waste products from the blood and at the same time to maintain the essential water and electrolyte balances in the body is controlled in the nephron by the following renal functions: renal blood flow, glomerular filtration, tubular reabsorption, and tubular secretion. The physiology, laboratory testing, and associated pathology of these four functions are discussed in this chapter.

RENAL BLOOD FLOW

Blood is supplied to the kidney by the renal artery and enters the nephron through the afferent arteriole. It flows through the glomerulus and into the efferent arteriole. The ability of these arterioles to vary in size helps create the hydrostatic pressure differential important for glomerular filtration and maintain consistency of glomerular capillary pressure and renal blood flow within the glomerulus. Notice the smaller size of the efferent arteriole in Figure 2–2. This produces an increase in the glomerular capillary pressure. Before returning to the renal vein, the blood from the efferent arteriole enters the peritubular

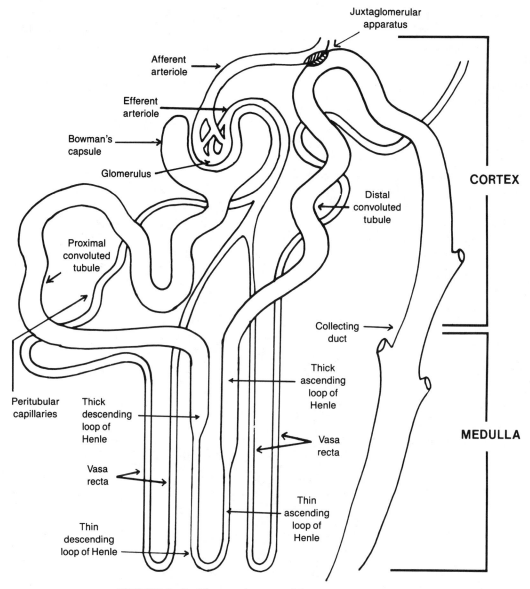

FIGURE 2–2. The nephron and its component parts.

capillaries and the vasa recta and flows slowly through the cortex and medulla of the kidney close to the tubules. The peritubular capillaries surround the proximal and distal convoluted tubules, providing for the immediate reabsorption of essential substances from the fluid in the proximal convoluted tubule and final adjustment of the urinary composition in the distal convoluted tubule. The vasa recta are located adjacent to the ascending and descending loops of Henle. It is in this area that the major exchanges of water and salts take place between the blood and the medullary interstitium. Removal of excess water and salts from the medullary interstitium by the blood flowing through the vasa recta maintains the osmotic gradient in the medulla that is necessary for renal concentration.

Based on an average body size of 1.73 square meters of surface, the total renal blood flow is approximately 1200 ml per minute, and the total renal plasma flow ranges from 600 to 700 ml per minute. Normal values for renal blood flow and renal function tests are dependent on body size. When dealing with sizes that vary gently from the average 1.73 square meters of surface, a correction must be calculated to determine whether the observed measurements represent normal function. This calculation is covered in the discussion on tests for glomerular filtration rate. Variations in normal values have also been published for different age groups and should be taken into consideration when evaluating renal function studies.

GLOMERULAR FILTRATION

Blood from the afferent arteriole enters the glomerulus within Bowman's capsule. The glomerulus consists of a coil of approximately eight capillary lobes referred to collectively as the capillary tuft. Although the glomerulus serves as a nonselective filter of plasma substances with molecular weights of less than 70,000, several factors influence the actual filtration process. These include the cellular structure of the capillary walls and Bowman's capsule, hydrostatic and oncotic pressures, and the feedback mechanisms of the renin-angiotensin system and aldosterone. Figure 2–3 provides a diagrammatic view of the glomerular areas influenced by these factors.

Plasma filtrate must pass through three cellular layers: the capillary wall membrane, the basement membrane (basal lamina), and the visceral epithelium of Bowman's cap-

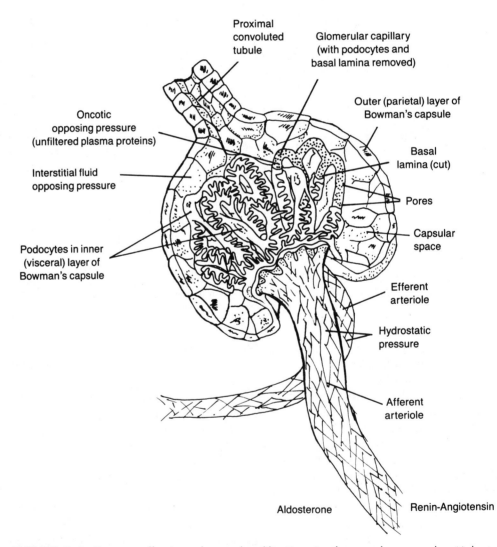

FIGURE 2–3. Factors affecting glomerular filtration in the renal corpuscle. (Adapted from Spence, A and Mason, E: Human Anatomy and Physiology. Benjamin/Cummings Publishing, Menlo Park, CA, 1987.)

sule. The endothelial cells of the capillary wall differ from those in other capillaries by containing pores and are referred to as fenestrated. The pores increase capillary permeability but do not allow the passage of large molecules and blood cells. Further restriction of large molecules occurs as the filtrate passes through the basement membrane and the thin membranes covering the filtration slits formed by the intertwining foot processes of the visceral epithelial podocytes (see Fig. 2–3).

As mentioned earlier, filtration is enhanced by the presence of hydrostatic pressure created by the smaller size of the efferent arteriole and the glomerular capillaries. This pressure is necessary to overcome the opposition of pressures from the fluid within Bowman's capsule and the colloidal pressure of unfiltered plasma proteins in the glomerular capillaries. By increasing or decreasing the size of the afferent arteriole, an autoregulatory mechanism within the kidney maintains the glomerular blood pressure at a relatively constant rate regardless of fluctuations in systemic blood pressure. Dilation of the afferent arterioles when blood pressure drops prevents a marked decrease in blood flowing through the kidney, thus preventing a rise in the blood level of toxic waste products.

Additional influence on the flow of blood through the kidney is provided by the renin-angiotensin system and aldosterone, which are activated in response to changes in blood flow to the kidney sensed by the macula densa in the juxtamedullary apparatus (see Fig. 2–2). The hormone aldosterone is secreted by the adrenal cortex and increases the reabsorption of sodium from the glomerular filtrate. Renin, an enzyme that is produced in the kidney when blood pressure levels decline, causes the production of aldosterone, which increases the reabsorption of sodium. This results in water retention, which increases extracellular fluid volume and intravascular pressure. As systemic pressure increases, production of renin is decreased, thus producing a decrease in angiotensin and aldosterone levels.

As a result of the above glomerular mechanisms, every minute approximately 120 ml of water containing low-molecular-weight substances are filtered through the 2 million glomeruli. Because this filtration is nonselective, the only difference between the compositions of the filtrate and the plasma is the absence of plasma protein, any protein-bound substances, and cells. Analysis of the fluid as it leaves the glomerulus shows the filtrate to have a specific gravity of 1.010 and confirms that it is chemically an ultrafiltrate of plasma. This information provides a useful baseline for evaluating the renal mechanisms involved in converting the plasma ultrafiltrate into the final urinary product.

TUBULAR REABSORPTION

It is obvious that the body cannot lose 120 ml of water containing essential substances every minute. Therefore, when the plasma ultrafiltrate enters the proximal convoluted tubule, the kidney, through cellular transport mechanisms, begins reabsorbing these essential substances and water. The cellular mechanisms involved in tubular reabsorption are termed active and passive transport. For active transport to occur, the substance to be reabsorbed must combine with a carrier protein contained in the membranes of the renal tubular cells. The electrochemical energy created by this interaction transfers the substance across the cell membranes and back into the blood stream. Active transport is responsible for the reabsorption of glucose, amino acids, and salts in the proximal convoluted tubule and the reabsorption of chloride in the ascending loop of Henle and sodium in the distal convoluted tubule. Passive transport is the movement of molecules across a membrane as a result of differences in their concentration or electrical potential on opposite sides of the membrane. These physical differences are called gradients. Passive reabsorption of water takes place in all parts of the nephron except the ascending loop of Henle, the walls of which are impermeable to water. Urea is passively reabsorbed in the proximal convoluted tubule and the ascending loop of Henle, and passive reabsorption of sodium accompanies the active transport of chloride in the ascending loop of Henle.[30]

Active transport, like passive transport, can be influenced by the concentration of the substance being transported. When the plasma concentration of a substance that is normally completely reabsorbed reaches an abnormally high level, the filtrate concentration exceeds the maximal reabsorptive capacity (Tm) of the tubules, and the substance begins appearing in the urine. The plasma concentration at which active transport stops is termed the "renal threshold." For glucose, the renal threshold is 160 to 180 mg per dl, and glycosuria occurs when the plasma concentration reaches this level. Knowledge of the renal threshold and the plasma concentration can be used to distinguish between excess solute filtration and renal tubular damage.

RENAL CONCENTRATION

Active transport of over two thirds of the filtered sodium out of the proximal convoluted tubule is accompanied by the passive reabsorption of an equal amount of water. Therefore, as can be seen in Figure 2–4, the fluid leaving the proximal convoluted tubule still maintains the same concentration as the ultrafiltrate.

Renal concentration begins in the descending and ascending loops of Henle, where the filtrate is exposed to the high osmotic gradient (salt concentration) of the renal medulla. Water is removed by osmosis in the descending loop of Henle, and sodium and chloride are reabsorbed in the ascending loop of Henle. Excessive reabsorption of water as the filtrate passes through the highly concentrated medulla is prevented by the water-impermeable walls of the ascending loop. This selective reabsorption process is called the countercurrent mechanism and serves to maintain the osmotic gradient of the me-

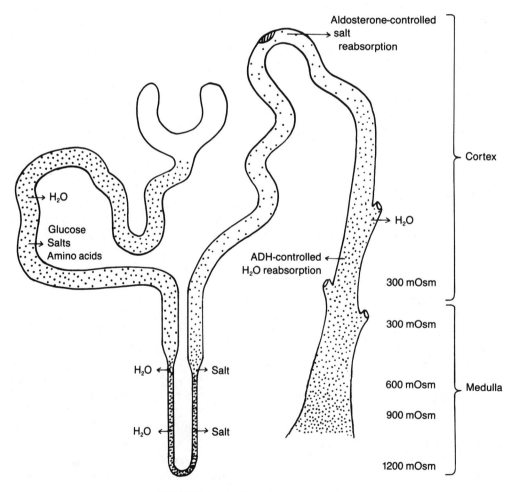

FIGURE 2–4. Renal concentration.

dulla. The sodium and chloride leaving the filtrate in the ascending loop prevent dilution of the medullary interstitium by the water reabsorbed from the descending loop. Maintenance of this osmotic gradient is essential for the final concentration of the filtrate when it reaches the collecting duct.

Notice in Figure 2–4 that the actual concentration of the filtrate leaving the ascending loop of Henle is quite low due to the reabsorption of salt and not water in that part of the tubule. Reabsorption of sodium continues in the distal convoluted tubule, but it is now under control of the hormone aldosterone, which regulates reabsorption in response to the body's need for sodium.

Final concentration of the filtrate through the reabsorption of water begins in the late distal convoluted tubule and continues in the collecting duct. Reabsorption is dependent on the osmotic gradient in the medulla and the hormone vasopressin (antidiuretic hormone [ADH]). One would expect that as the dilute filtrate comes in contact with the higher osmotic concentration in the medullary interstitium, passive reabsorption of water would occur. However, the process is controlled by the presence or absence of ADH, which renders the walls of the distal convoluted tubule and collecting duct permeable or impermeable to water. A high level of ADH increases permeability, resulting in increased reabsorption of water and a low-volume, concentrated urine. Likewise, absence of ADH renders the walls impermeable to water, resulting in a large volume of dilute urine. Just as the production of aldosterone is controlled by the body's sodium concentration, production of ADH is determined by the state of body hydration. Therefore, the chemical balance in the body is actually the final determinant of urine volume and concentration.

TUBULAR SECRETION

In contrast to tubular reabsorption, in which substances are removed from the glomerular filtrate and returned to the blood, tubular secretion involves the passage of substances from the blood in the peritubular capillaries to the tubular filtrate (Fig. 2–5). Tubular secretion serves two major functions: elimination of waste products not filtered by the glomerulus, and regulation of the acid-base balance in the body through the secretion of hydrogen ions. Many foreign substances, such as medications, cannot be filtered by the glomerulus because they are bound to plasma proteins. However, when these protein-bound substances enter the peritubular capillaries, they develop a strong affinity for the tubular cells and dissociate from their carrier proteins, which results in their transportation into the filtrate by the tubular cells. The major site for removal of these nonfiltered substances is the proximal convoluted tubule.

To maintain the normal blood pH of 7.4 it is necessary to buffer and to eliminate the excess acid formed by dietary intake and body metabolism. The buffering capacity of the blood is dependent on bicarbonate ions, which are readily filtered by the glomerulus and must be expediently returned to the blood to maintain the proper pH. As shown in Figure 2–6, the secretion of hydrogen ions by the renal tubular cells prevents the filtered bicarbonate from being excreted in the urine and causes the return of a bicarbonate ion to the plasma. This process provides for almost 100 percent reabsorption of filtered bicarbonate and occurs primarily in the proximal convoluted tubule.

The actual excretion of excess hydrogen ions is also dependent on tubular secretion. Figures 2–7 and 2–8 diagram the two primary methods for hydrogen ion excretion in the urine. In Figure 2–7, the secreted hydrogen ion combines with a filtered phosphate ion instead of a bicarbonate ion and is excreted rather than reabsorbed. Additional excretion of hydrogen ions is accomplished through their reaction with ammonia produced and secreted by the cells of the distal convoluted tubule, as shown in Figure 2–8. The resulting ammonium ion is excreted in the urine.

All three of these processes are occurring simultaneously at rates determined by the acid-base balance in the body. A disruption in these secretory functions can result in the disorder called metabolic acidosis.

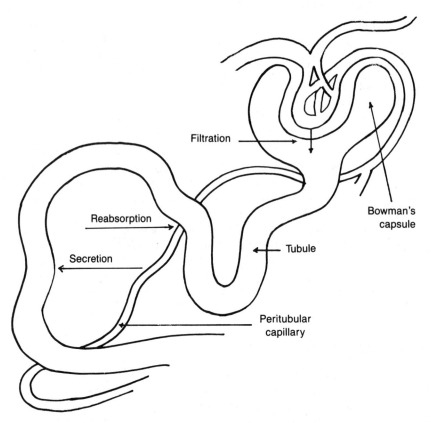

FIGURE 2–5. The movement of substances in the nephron.

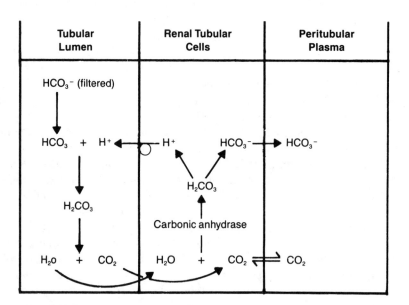

FIGURE 2–6. Mechanism by which filtered bicarbonate is reabsorbed. (From Vander,[30] with permission.)

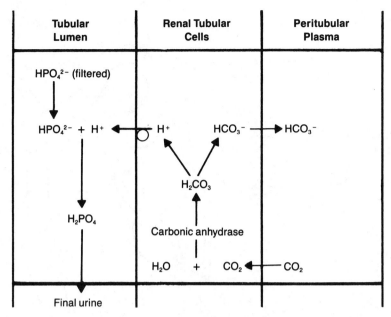

FIGURE 2–7. Reaction of secreted hydrogen ion with filtered phosphate. (From Vander,[30] with permission.)

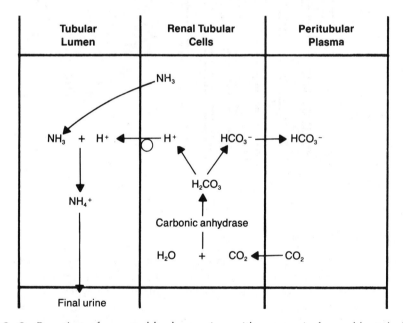

FIGURE 2–8. Reaction of secreted hydrogen ion with ammonia formed by tubular cells. (From Vander,[30] with permission.)

RENAL FUNCTION TESTS

As can be seen from the brief review of renal physiology, there are many metabolic functions and chemical interactions to be evaluated through laboratory tests of renal function. Figure 2–9 relates the parts of the nephron to the laboratory tests used to assess their function.

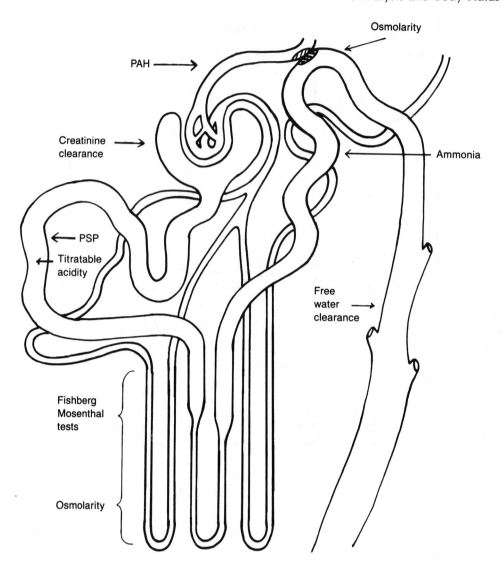

FIGURE 2–9. The relationship of nephron areas to renal function tests.

GLOMERULAR FILTRATION TESTS

The standard test used to measure the filtering capacity of the glomeruli is the clearance test. As its name implies, a clearance test measures the rate at which the kidneys are able to remove (to clear) a filterable substance from the blood. To ensure that glomerular filtration is being accurately measured, the substance analyzed must be one that is neither reabsorbed nor secreted by the tubules. Furthermore, the stability of the substance in urine during a possible 24-hour collection period, the consistency of the plasma level, the substance's availability to the body, and the ease of chemical analysis of the substance are also factors that must be taken into consideration in the selection of a clearance test substance.

Clearance Tests

The earliest glomerular filtration tests measured urea because of its presence in all urine specimens and the existence of proven methods of chemical analysis. Because approximately 40 percent of the filtered urea is reabsorbed, normal values were adjusted to reflect the reabsorption, and patients were hydrated to produce a urine flow of 2 ml per minute to ensure that no more than 40 percent of the urea was reabsorbed. At the present time, the use of urea as a test substance for glomerular filtration has been almost entirely replaced by the measurement of either creatinine, inulin, β_2 microglobulin, or radioisotopes.

Inulin, a polymer of fructose, is an extremely stable substance that is not reabsorbed or secreted by the tubules. However, it is not a normal body constituent and must be infused at a constant rate throughout the testing period. A test that requires an infused substance is termed an exogenous procedure and is seldom the method of choice if a suitable test substance is already present in the body (endogenous procedure). Therefore, inulin has not been routinely used for glomerular filtration testing.

The development of simplified procedures measuring the plasma disappearance of infused substances, thereby eliminating the need for urine collection, has enhanced interest in exogenous procedures.[5, 29] Injection of radionucleotides provides not only a method for determining glomerular filtration through the plasma disappearance of the radioactive material but also enables visualization of the filtration in one or both kidneys.[7]

Good correlation between the glomerular filtration rate and plasma levels of β_2 microglobulin has recently been demonstrated. β_2 microglobulin (molecular weight 11,800) dissociates from human leukocyte antigens at a constant rate and is rapidly removed from the plasma by glomerular filtration. Sensitive methods utilizing radioimmunoassay and enzyme immunoassay are available for the measurement of β_2 microglobulin.[26] A rise in the plasma level of β_2 microglobulin has been shown to be a more sensitive indicator of a decrease in glomerular filtration rate than the creatinine clearance. However, the test is not reliable in patients who have a history of immunologic disorders or malignancy.[23]

Currently, routine laboratory measurements of glomerular filtration rate employ creatinine as the test substance. Creatinine, a waste product of muscle metabolism that is normally found at a relatively constant level in the blood, provides the laboratory with an endogenous procedure for evaluating glomerular function. The use of creatinine has several disadvantages not found with inulin, and careful consideration should be given to them:

1. Some creatinine is secreted by the tubules, and secretion increases as blood levels rise.
2. Chromogens present in human plasma react in the chemical analysis. However, their presence may help counteract the falsely elevated rates caused by tubular secretion.
3. Urinary creatinine will be broken down by bacteria if specimens are kept at room temperature for extended periods of time.[22]
4. A heavy meat diet consumed during collection of a 24-hour urine specimen will influence the results if the plasma specimen is drawn prior to the collection period.[17]
5. Measurement of creatinine clearance is not a reliable indicator in patients suffering from muscle-wasting diseases.[27]

Because of these drawbacks, abnormal results may be followed up with more sophisticated tests, but the creatinine clearance test can provide the routine clinical laboratory with a method to screen the glomerular filtration rate.[12] Measurement of plasma creatinine under controlled conditions also can be used to monitor renal function.[25]

Calculations

By far the greatest source of error in any clearance procedure is the use of improperly timed urine specimens. The importance of using an accurately timed specimen, as described in chapter 1, will become evident as we now discuss the calculations involved in converting isolated laboratory measurements to glomerular filtration rate. The glomerular filtration rate is reported in milliliters per minute; therefore, it is necessary to determine the number of milliliters of plasma from which the clearance substance (creatinine) is completely removed during a 1-minute period. To calculate this information, one must know urine volume in ml per minute (V), urine creatinine concentration in mg per dl (U), and plasma creatinine concentration in mg per dl (P).

The urine volume is calculated by dividing the number of milliliters in the specimen by the number of minutes used to collect the specimen.

Example: Calculate the urine volume (V) for a 2-hour specimen measuring 240 milliliters:

$$2 \text{ hours} \times 60 \text{ minutes} = 120 \text{ minutes}$$

$$\frac{240 \text{ ml}}{120 \text{ min}} = 2 \text{ ml/min} \qquad V = 2 \text{ ml/min}$$

The plasma and urine concentrations are determined by chemical testing. The standard formula used to calculate the milliliters of plasma cleared per minute (C) is:

$$C = \frac{UV}{P}$$

This formula is derived as follows: The milliliters of plasma cleared per minute (C) times the milligrams per deciliter of plasma creatinine (P) must equal the milligrams per deciliter of urine creatinine (U) times the urine volume in milliliters per minute (V), because all of the filtered creatinine will appear in the urine. Therefore,

$$CP = UV \quad \text{and} \quad C = \frac{UV}{P}$$

Example: Using urine creatinine of 120 mg/dl (U), plasma creatinine of 1.0 mg/dl (P), and urine volume of 60 ml obtained from a 1-hour specimen (V), calculate the glomerular filtration rate (creatinine clearance) (C):

$$V = \frac{60 \text{ ml}}{60 \text{ min}} = 1 \text{ ml/min}$$

$$C = \frac{120 \text{ mg/dl (U)} \times 1 \text{ ml/min (V)}}{1.0 \text{ mg/dl (P)}} = 120 \text{ ml/min}$$

By analyzing this calculation and referring to Figure 2–10, we can see that at a 1 mg per dl concentration, each milliliter of plasma contains 0.01 mg creatinine. Therefore, to ar-

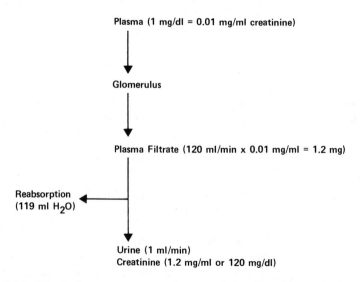

Plasma (1 mg/dl = 0.01 mg/ml creatinine)

Glomerulus

Plasma Filtrate (120 ml/min x 0.01 mg/ml = 1.2 mg)

Reabsorption
(119 ml H_2O)

Urine (1 ml/min)
Creatinine (1.2 mg/ml or 120 mg/dl)

FIGURE 2–10. A diagram representing creatinine filtration and excretion.

rive at a urine concentration of 120 mg per dl (1.2 mg per ml), it would be necessary to clear 120 ml of plasma. Notice also that although the filtrate volume is reduced, the amount of creatinine in the filtrate does not change.

Knowing that in the average person (1.73 square meter body surface) the approximate amount of plasma filtrate produced per minute is 120 ml, it is not surprising that normal creatinine clearance values approach 120 ml per min (men, 107 to 139 ml per min; women, 87 to 107 ml per min). The normal plasma creatinine is 0.5 to 1.5 mg per dl. These normal values take into account variations in size and muscle mass. However, values are considerably lower in older people, and an adjustment may also have to be made to the calculation when dealing with body sizes that deviate greatly from 1.73 square meters of surface, such as in children. To adjust a clearance for body size, the formula is:

$$C = \frac{UV}{P} \times \frac{1.73}{A}$$

with A being the actual body size in square meters of surface. The actual body size may be calculated as:

$$\log A = (0.425 \times \log weight) + (0.725 \times \log height) - 2.144$$

or it may be obtained from the nomogram shown in Figure 2–11.

Clinical Significance

When interpreting the results of a creatinine clearance test, one must keep in mind that the glomerular filtration rate is determined not only by the number of functioning nephrons but also by the functional capacity of these nephrons. In other words, even though one half of the available nephrons may be nonfunctional, a change in the glomerular filtration rate will not occur if the remaining nephrons double their filtering capacity. This is evidenced by those persons who lead normal lives with only one kidney. Therefore, although the creatinine clearance is a frequently requested laboratory procedure, its value does not lie in the detection of early renal disease. It is used, instead, to determine the extent of nephron damage in known cases of renal disease, to monitor the effectiveness of treatment designed to prevent further nephron damage, and to determine the feasibility of administering medications, which can build up to dangerous blood levels if the glomerular filtration rate is markedly reduced.

TUBULAR REABSORPTION TESTS

Whereas measurement of the glomerular filtration rate is not a useful indication of early renal disease, the loss of tubular reabsorption capability is often the first function affected in renal disease. This is not surprising when one considers the complexity of the tubular reabsorption process.

Tests to determine the ability of the tubules to reabsorb the essential salts and water that have been nonselectively filtered by the glomerulus are collectively termed concentration tests. As mentioned earlier, the ultrafiltrate that enters the tubules has a specific gravity of 1.010; therefore, after reabsorption one would expect the final urine product to be more concentrated. However, from our experience in performing routine urinalysis, we know that many specimens do not have a specific gravity higher than 1.010; yet there is no renal disease present. This is because urine concentration is largely determined by the body's state of hydration, and the normal kidney will reabsorb only the amount of water necessary to preserve an adequate supply of body water.

As can be seen in Figure 2–12, both specimens contain the same amount of solute; however, the urine density (specific gravity) of Patient A will be higher. Therefore, control of fluid intake must be incorporated into laboratory tests that measure the concentrating ability of the kidney. Various methods are available to provide water deprivation and

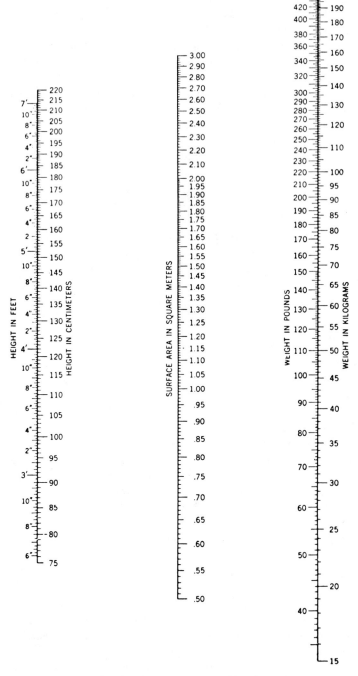

FIGURE 2–11. A nomogram for the determination of body surface area. (From Boothby, WM and Sandiford, RB: Nomogram for determination of body surface area. N Engl J Med 185:337, 1921, with permission.)

controlled specimens for analysis. Two well-known procedures are the Fishberg and Mosenthal tests.

Fishberg Test

In the Fishberg concentration test, the patient eats a normal breakfast and then consumes no more fluid until 8 AM the next morning. At that time, the patient collects a urine speci-

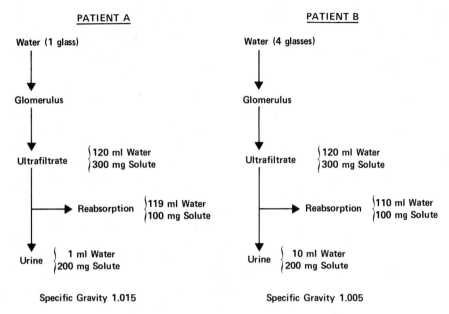

FIGURE 2–12. The effect of hydration on specific gravity.

men and then remains in bed for 1 hour, collects another specimen, resumes normal activity for 1 hour, and collects a third specimen. The specific gravity of at least one of these specimens should be 1.026 or higher. A simplified version of the Fishberg procedure that is routinely used in many laboratories requires the patient to restrict fluids either with or immediately following the evening meal and then to collect specimens at 7 AM, 8 AM, and 9 AM the following morning. Each specimen is tested for specific gravity, and at least one specimen should measure 1.022 or higher. With both of these procedures, the first specimen voided may not have the highest specific gravity, inasmuch as nocturnal diuresis in some patients produces a diluted first specimen.

Mosenthal Test

The Mosenthal test allows the patient to maintain a normal diet and fluid intake; however, urine is collected over a 24-hour period. After emptying the bladder at 8 AM, the patient is instructed to collect all urine passed between 8 AM and 8 PM in one container and to collect all urine passed between 8 PM and 8 AM in a second container. In the laboratory, both specimens are measured and tested for specific gravity. Persons with normal concentrating ability will produce a day specimen (8 AM to 8 PM) with a higher volume and lower specific gravity than the night specimen (8 PM to 8 AM).

EXAMPLE

Normal

8 AM – 8 PM specimen
Specific gravity 1.015
Volume 1000 ml

8 PM – 8 AM specimen
Specific gravity 1.025
Volume 400 ml

Abnormal

8 AM – 8 PM specimen
Specific gravity 1.015
Volume 400 ml

8 PM – 8 AM specimen
Specific gravity 1.011
Volume 500 ml

Osmolarity

Although the simplicity of the specific gravity measurements employed in the Fishberg and Mosenthal tests is convenient for routine clinical use, a more accurate evaluation of renal concentrating ability can be obtained by measuring serum and urine osmolarity. Specific gravity (measured by urinometry) depends on the number of particles present in a solution and the density of these particles; whereas osmolarity is affected only by the number of particles present. When evaluating renal concentration ability, the substances of interest are small molecules, primarily sodium (molecular weight, 23) and chloride (molecular weight, 35.5). However, urea (molecular weight, 60), which is of no importance to this evaluation, will contribute more to the specific gravity than the sodium and chloride molecules. Because all three of these molecules contribute equally to the osmolarity of the specimen, a more representative measure of renal concentrating ability can be obtained by measuring osmolarity. Comparisons between refractometry, reagent strips, and osmolarity for monitoring fluid balance in neonates have shown that osmolarity provides much more reliable information.[1, 4]

An osmole is defined as 1 gram molecular weight of a substance divided by the number of particles into which it dissociates.[6] A nonionizing substance such as glucose (molecular weight, 180) contains 180 grams per osmole; whereas sodium chloride (NaCl) (molecular weight, 58.5), if completely dissociated, contains 29.25 grams per osmole. Just as we have the terms molality and molarity, we have osmolality and osmolarity. An osmolal solution of glucose has 180 grams of glucose dissolved in 1 kilogram of solvent, and an osmolar solution has 180 grams of glucose dissolved in 1 liter of solvent. In the clinical laboratory, the terms are used interchangeably, inasmuch as the difference under normal temperature conditions with water as the solvent is minimal. The unit of measure used in the clinical laboratory is the milliosmole (mOsm), because it is not practical when dealing with body fluids to use a measurement as large as the osmole (23 grams of sodium per liter or kilogram). The osmolarity of a solution can be determined by measuring a property that is mathematically related to the number of particles in the solution (colligative property) and comparing this value with the value obtained from the pure solvent. Solute dissolved in solvent causes the following changes in colligative properties: lower freezing point, higher boiling point, increased osmotic pressure, and lower vapor pressure.

Because water is the solvent in both urine and plasma, it is possible to determine the number of particles present in a sample by comparing a colligative property value of the sample with that of pure water. Clinical laboratory instruments are available to measure freezing point depression and vapor pressure depression.

Clinical Osmometers

Measurement of freezing point depression was the first principle incorporated into clinical osmometers, and many instruments employing this technique are available. These osmometers determine the freezing point of a solution by supercooling a measured amount of sample to approximately $-7°C$. The supercooled sample is then vibrated to produce crystallization of water in the solution. The heat of fusion produced by the crystallizing water temporarily raises the temperature of the solution to its freezing point. A temperature-sensitive probe measures this temperature rise, and the information is transferred by means of a Wheatstone bridge to a galvanometer and converted into milliosmoles.[31] Conversion is made possible by the fact that 1 mole (1000 mOsm) of a nonionizing substance dissolved in 1 kilogram of water is known to lower the freezing point $1.86°C$. Therefore, by comparing the freezing point depression of a solution containing ionizing and nonionizing substances with the $-1.86°C$ depression of a solution of nonionizing substance, the number of milliosmoles in the mixed solution can be determined. For example, one mole of NaCL dissolved in one kilogram of water depresses the freezing point $-3.46°C$. Calculate the osmolarity of the solution:

$$\frac{1000 \, mOsm}{-1.86} = \frac{X \, mOsm}{-3.46}$$

$$-1.86X = -3.46 \times 1000$$

$$X = 1860 \, mOsm$$

Clinical osmometers use solutions of NaCl as their reference standards because a solution of partially ionized substances is more representative of urine and plasma composition. Standards of both low and high concentration can be prepared in the manner shown above.

The newest addition to clinical osmometry is called the vapor pressure osmometer. However, the actual measurement performed is the dew point (temperature at which water vapor condenses to a liquid). The depression of dew-point temperature by solute parallels the decrease in vapor pressure, thereby providing a measure of this colligative property.

Samples are absorbed into small filter paper disks that are placed in a sealed chamber containing a temperature-sensitive thermocoupler. As water condenses in the chamber and on the thermocoupler, the heat of condensation produced raises the temperature of the thermocoupler to the dew-point temperature. This dew point temperature is proportional to the vapor pressure from the evaporating sample. Temperatures are compared with those of the NaCl standards and converted into milliosmols. The vapor pressure osmometer uses microsamples of less than 0.01 ml, therefore care must be taken to prevent any evaporation of the sample prior to testing. Correlation studies have shown more variation with vapor pressure osmometers, stressing the necessity of careful technique.[19]

Clinical Significance

Factors that should be taken into consideration because of their influence on true osmolarity readings include lipemic serum and the presence of lactic acid or volatile substances, such as ethanol, in the specimen. In lipemic serum, the displacement of serum water by insoluble lipids produces erroneous results with both vapor pressure and freezing-point osmometers. Falsely elevated values owing to the formation of lactic acid also will occur with both methods if serum samples are not separated or refrigerated within 20 minutes.[21] Vapor pressure osmometers will not detect the presence of volatile substances,[21] inasmuch as they become part of the solvent phase; however, measurements performed on similar specimens using freezing-point osmometers will be elevated. Comparisons of serum osmolarities run on cryoscopic and vapor pressure osmometers have been suggested as a method for rapid screening of comatose patients for alcohol ingestion.[9, 31] Major clinical uses of osmolarity include initial evaluation of renal concentrating ability, monitoring the course of renal disease, monitoring fluid and electrolyte therapy, establishing the differential diagnosis of hypernatremia and hyponatremia and polyuria, and evaluating the secretion of and renal response to ADH.[24]

Normal serum osmolarity values are between 275 and 300 mOsm. Normal values for urine osmolarity are difficult to establish, because factors such as diet and exercise can greatly influence the urine concentration and values can range between 50 and 1400 mOsm.[22] Therefore, it is often necessary to measure both serum and urine osmolarity and to evaluate the ratio obtained from the two readings. Under normal random conditions, the ratio of urine to serum osmolarity should be at least 1:1; after controlled fluid intake, it should reach 3:1. Determination of the urine-to-serum osmolarity ratio, in conjunction with procedures such as controlled fluid intake and injection of ADH, is used to differentiate whether diabetes insipidus is due to decreased ADH production or the inability of the renal tubules to respond to ADH, to aid in the identification of tumors that produce ADH-like substances, and to determine the underlying causes of apparent renal pathology.[2] Tests to measure the ADH concentration in plasma and urine directly are available for difficult diagnostic cases.[28]

Free Water Clearance

When dealing with difficult diagnostic problems, it may become necessary to expand the urine-to-serum osmolarity ratio further by performing the analyses using a timed urine specimen and calculating the free water clearance. The free water clearance is determined by first calculating the osmolar clearance using the standard clearance formula of

$$C_{osm} = \frac{U_{osm} \times V}{P_{osm}}$$

and then subtracting the osmolar clearance value from the urine volume.

Example: Using urine osmolarity of 600 mOsm (U), urine volume of 2 ml/min (V), and plasma osmolarity of 300 mOsm (P), calculate the free water clearance:

$$C_{osm} = \frac{600\,(U) \times 2\,(V)}{300\,(P)} = 4.0\,ml/min$$

$$C_{H_{2}0} = 2\,(V) - 4.0\,(C_{osm}) = -2.0$$

Calculation of the osmolar clearance tells how much water must be cleared each minute to produce a urine with the same osmolarity as the plasma. Remember that the ultrafiltrate contains the same osmolarity as the plasma; therefore, the osmotic differences found in the urine are the result of renal concentrating and diluting mechanisms. By comparing the osmolar clearance with the actual urine volume excreted per minute, it can be determined whether the water being excreted is more or less than the amount needed to maintain an osmolarity the same as the ultrafiltrate. The above calculation shows a free water clearance of -2.0, indicating that less than the necessary amount of water is being excreted and that renal concentration is taking place. If the value had been zero, no renal concentration or dilution would be taking place; likewise, if the value had been $+2.0$, renal dilution would be occurring.[22] Therefore, calculation of the free water clearance can be used to determine the amount and type of work being done by the tubules.

TUBULAR SECRETION AND RENAL BLOOD FLOW TESTS

Tests to measure tubular secretion of nonfiltered substances and renal blood flow are closely related inasmuch as total renal blood flow through the nephron must be measured by a substance that is secreted rather than filtered through the glomerulus. An abnormal result may be caused either by impaired tubular secretory ability or inadequate presentation of the substance to the capillaries due to decreased renal blood flow. Therefore, understanding of the principles and limitations of the tests and correlation with other clinical data is important in their interpretation. The two tests most commonly associated with tubular secretion and renal blood flow are the phenolsulfonphthalein (PSP) test and the p-aminohippuric acid (PAH) test. Both tests rely on tubular secretion for the measurement of renal blood flow.

PSP TEST

Phenolsulfonphthalein is a dye. When it is injected into the blood stream, approximately 94 percent of the dye binds to the plasma proteins. The protein-bound dye cannot be filtered by the glomerulus and must be removed by tubular secretion. PSP dye is secreted in the proximal convoluted tubule, where the dye has a stronger affinity for the cells lining the tubule than it does for the plasma proteins; therefore, it dissociates from the plasma proteins and is secreted into the filtrate by the cells of the proximal convoluted tubule.

The PSP test is performed by injecting 6 mg of phenolsulfonphthalein dye into a well-hydrated patient; collecting urine specimens at 15, 30, 60, and 120 minutes postinjection; and measuring the amount of dye excreted in each specimen. Measurement of the dye concentration is based on the principle that phenolsulfonphthalein produces a pink color in alkaline solutions. The urine specimens are made alkaline with sodium hydroxide and diluted to a uniform volume with distilled water, and the intensity of the pink color is compared with standards of known concentration using a spectrophotometer. Substances that produce a cloudy specimen, such as blood and amorphous crystals, will interfere with the spectrophotometer readings and should be removed by centrifugation prior to performing the test. Patients should also be cautioned to avoid foods that produce highly pigmented urine and to refrain from taking medications for 24 hours prior to the test. [3]

Accurate timing and collection of the specimens are critical because normal values are based on the percentage of dye excreted in the four time periods. The 15-minute specimen is the most informative, because as given enough time, even poorly functioning kidneys will excrete the dye. This specimen normally contains about 35 percent of the dye. By the end of the first hour, approximately 60 percent of the dye has been excreted: at the end of 2 hours, 75 percent. Values below 25 percent in the 15-minute specimen indicate impaired renal function. Even though the method of dye removal is tubular secretion and the PSP test is often referred to as a secretion test, the defective function is often renal blood flow. This is because the small amount of diluted dye presented to the tubules will be secreted unless the cells are severely damaged. Therefore, failure to excrete an acceptable amount of the dye in the 15-minute specimen by a patient without severe renal disease must be attributed to inadequate renal blood flow, which causes a delay in the presentation of the dye to the tubule cells.

PAH Test

The ease by which the PSP test can be performed has made it a popular screening test for renal blood flow. However, because the dye is not completely removed from the blood during a single pass through the kidney, it cannot be used to determine the actual blood flow in milliliters per minute. To measure the exact amount of blood flowing through the kidney, it is necessary to use a substance that is completely removed from the blood (plasma) each time it comes in contact with functional renal tissue. The principle is the same as in the clearance test for glomerular filtration. However, to ensure measurement of the blood flow through the entire nephron, the substance must be removed from the blood primarily in the peritubular capillaries, rather than being removed when the blood reaches the glomerulus. Although it has the disadvantage of being exogenous, the chemical p-aminohippurate (PAH) meets the criteria needed to measure renal blood flow. It is a nontoxic substance that binds less strongly to plasma proteins than PSP dye, which permits its complete removal as the blood passes through the peritubular capillaries. Except for a small amount of PAH that does not come in contact with functional renal tissue, all of plasma PAH is secreted by the proximal convoluted tubule. The amount of PAH excreted in the urine will be determined by the volume of plasma flowing through the kidneys. The standard clearance formula

$$C_{PAH}(\text{ml/min}) = \frac{U \text{ (mg/dl PAH)} \times V \text{ (ml/min urine)}}{P \text{ (mg/dl PAH)}}$$

can be used to calculate the effective renal plasma flow. Normal values for the effective renal plasma flow range from 600 to 700 ml per minute, making the average renal blood flow about 1200 ml per minute. Notice that the actual measurement is renal plasma flow rather than renal blood flow, because the PAH is contained only in the plasma portion of the blood. Also, the term "effective" is included because approximately 8 percent of the renal blood flow does not come into contact with the functional renal tissue. [10]

The PAH test is not routinely performed in the clinical laboratory, and patients are referred to specialized renal laboratories or nuclear medicine departments. Procedures utilizing radioactive hippurate can determine renal blood flow by measuring the plasma disappearance of a single radioactive injection and at the same time provide visualization of the blood flowing through the kidneys. [7, 29]

TITRATABLE ACIDITY AND URINARY AMMONIA

As discussed earlier, the ability of the kidney to produce an acid urine is dependent on the tubular secretion of hydrogen ions and production and secretion of ammonia by the cells of the distal convoluted tubule. A normal person excretes approximately 70 mEq of acid per day in the form of either titratable acid (H^+) or ammonium ions (NH_4^+).

The inability to produce an acid urine in the presence of metabolic acidosis is called renal tubular acidosis and may result from impaired tubular secretion of hydrogen ions or defects in ammonia production and secretion. Measurement of urinary titratable acidity and urinary ammonia can be used to determine the defective function. The tests can be run simultaneously on either fresh or toluene-preserved urine specimens collected at 2-hour intervals from patients who have been primed with an acid load consisting of oral ammonium chloride. By titrating the amount of free H^+ (titratable acidity) and then the total acidity of the specimen, the ammonium concentration can be calculated as the difference between the titratable acidity and the total acidity.[8] In a normal person, approximately two thirds of the excreted acid is ammonium ion and one third is in the form of titratable acid. Variations in the ratio, along with a decrease in total acid excretion, can then be analyzed to determine whether the patient's problem is due to lack of hydrogen ion secretion or decreased ammonia production.

RENAL DISEASES

Although disease states throughout the body can affect renal function and produce abnormalities in the urinalysis, abnormal results are frequently associated with disorders directly affecting the kidney. A basic discussion of the major renal diseases—including possible causes, clinical symptoms, associated pathology, and laboratory findings (Table 2–1)—is presented at this point to enable laboratory personnel to better understand the significance of test results in these conditions.

Acute Glomerulonephritis

In general, glomerulonephritis refers to a sterile inflammatory process that affects the glomerulus and is associated with the finding of blood, protein, and casts in the urine.[11] Acute glomerulonephritis, as the name implies, is a disease characterized by the rapid onset of symptoms consistent with damage to the glomerular membrane. It is most frequently seen in children and young adults following respiratory tract infections caused by certain strains of group A streptococci. During the course of the infection, these nephrogenic strains of streptococci are believed to form immune complexes with circulating antibodies and become deposited on the glomerular membrane, resulting in damage to the integrity of the membrane. Similar damage also can be produced by exposure to nephrotoxic chemicals.[14] In most cases, successful management of the secondary complications—which include edema, hypertension, and electrolyte imbalance until the inflammation has subsided—will result in a permanent cure.

A more serious form of the disease, called crescentic (or rapidly progressive) glomerulonephritis, has a much poorer prognosis, often terminating in renal failure. Crescent formation by epithelial cells on the inside of Bowman's capsule and changes in the glomerular capillary tufts from fibrin deposition cause breakage of the capillary basement membrane, resulting in permanent damage to the glomeruli. Crescentic glomerulonephritis may also develop as a complication in other forms of glomerulonephritis or systemic diseases, such as systemic lupus erythematosus.

Primary urinalysis findings include marked hematuria, increased protein, and oliguria, accompanied by red blood cell casts, dysmorphic red blood cells, hyaline and granular casts, and white blood cells. As toxicity to the glomerular membrane subsides, the urinalysis results will return to normal, with the possible exception of microscopic hematuria that lasts until the membrane damage has been repaired. Blood urea nitrogen (BUN) may be elevated during the acute stages but, like the urinalysis, will return to normal unless the disease develops into crescentic glomerulonephritis. Demonstration of an elevated serum antistreptolysin O titer provides evidence that the disease is of streptococcal origin.

CHRONIC GLOMERULONEPHRITIS

The term chronic glomerulonephritis has been used to describe a variety of disorders that produce continual or permanent damage to the glomerulus. Classifications vary somewhat among authors but primarily include membranous, mesangiocapillary (or membranoproliferative) and focal glomerulonephritis, and minimal change disease. Currently, these conditions are categorized separately, and chronic glomerulonephritis is used to represent the end-stage result of persistent glomerular damage associated with irreversible loss of renal tissue and chronic renal failure.[16] Clinical symptoms include edema, hypertension, anemia, metabolic acidosis, and oliguria progressing to anuria. Examination of the urine in chronic glomerulonephritis reveals the presence of blood, protein, and many varieties of casts, including broad casts, and a specific gravity of 1.010, indicating a loss of renal concentrating ability and a decreased glomerular filtration rate. Blood urea nitrogen and creatinine are elevated, as are the serum phosphorus and potassium. Serum calcium levels are noticeably decreased.

Nephrotic Syndrome

The nephrotic syndrome is characterized by the appearance of massive proteinuria, edema, high levels of serum lipids, and low levels of serum albumin.[11] Circulatory disorders that affect the pressure and flow of blood to the kidney are one of the most frequent causes of the nephrotic syndrome, and it may occur as a complication in cases of glomerulonephritis. Changes in the permeability of the glomerular membrane permit the passage of high molecular weight proteins and lipids into the glomerular filtrate. Absorption of the lipid-containing proteins by the renal tubular cells followed by cellular sloughing produces the characteristic oval fat bodies and fatty casts seen in the sediment examination. Tubular damage, as well as glomerular damage, occurs, and the condition may progress to chronic renal failure.

Urinalysis observations include marked proteinuria, urinary fat droplets, oval fat bodies, renal tubular epithelial cells and casts, waxy and fatty casts, or, in general, a telescoped sediment.

Membranous Glomerulonephritis

The predominant characteristic of membranous glomerulonephritis is a pronounced thickening of the glomerular capillary basement membrane. In autoimmune diseases, such as systemic lupus erythematosus, deposition of immune complexes on the membrane produces the thickening. However, increased membrane epithelial cell production leading to membrane thickening occurs with secondary syphilis, Sjogren's syndrome, gold and mercury treatments, hepatitis B antigen, and malignancies. Many cases of unknown etiology also have been diagnosed.[14] As a rule, the disease progresses slowly, and remissions are frequent; but the patient may eventually develop a nephrotic syndrome.

Laboratory findings include microscopic hematuria and elevated urine protein excretion that may reach concentrations similar to those in the nephrotic syndrome. Demonstration of systemic lupus erythematosus or hepatitis B through blood tests can aid in the diagnosis.

Mesangiocapillary Glomerulonephritis

Sometimes referred to as membranoproliferative glomerulonephritis, this form of glomerulonephritis is characterized by two different alterations in the cellularity of the glomerulus and peripheral capillaries. Type I displays increased cellularity in the subendothelial cells of the mesangium; whereas type II displays extremely dense deposits in the glomerular basement membrane. Many of the patients are children, and the disease has a poor

TABLE 2–1. Laboratory Correlations in Renal Diseases[13–16]

DISEASE	ROUTINE URINALYSIS	MICROSCOPIC EXAMINATION	OTHER LABORATORY FINDINGS	REMARKS
Acute glomerulonephritis	Macroscopic hematuria Specific gravity ↑ Protein <5 g/day	RBCs RBC casts Granular casts WBCs	ASO titer ↑ GFR ↓ Sedrate ↑	Microscopic hematuria remains longer than proteinuria RBCs usually dysmorphic
Crescentic (rapidly progressive) glomerulonephritis	Macroscopic hematuria Protein	RBCs WBCs Granular casts	BUN ↑ Creatinine ↑ Fibrin degradation products ↑ GFR ↓ Cryoglobulins ↑	Oliguria RBCs usually dysmorphic
Chronic glomerulonephritis	Macroscopic hematuria Specific gravity 1.010 Protein	RBCs, dysmorphic WBCs All types of casts Broad casts	BUN ↑ Creatinine ↑ Serum phosphorus ↑ Serum calcium ↓	Oliguria or anuria Nocturia Anemia
Membranous glomerulonephritis	Blood Protein	RBCs Hyaline casts	Positive ANA Positive HB$_s$Ag	Microscopic hematuria
Mesangiocapillary (membranoproliferative) glomerulonephritis	Macroscopic hematuria Protein	RBCs RBC casts Other casts	BUN ↑ Creatinine ↑ Complement ↓	Hematuria may be microscopic Characteristics of the nephrotic syndrome may be present
Focal glomerulonephritis	Blood Protein	RBCs WBCs Fat droplets	Immune deposits on membrane	Macroscopic or microscopic hematuria

Disease	Physical/Chemical	Microscopic	Other Tests	Comments
Minimal change disease	Blood Protein	RBCs Oval fat bodies Fat droplets Hyaline casts Fatty casts	Serum protein ↓ Serum albumin ↓	Hematuria may be absent
Nephrotic syndrome	Protein	Oval fat bodies Fat droplets Generalized casts Waxy casts Fatty casts	Serum lipids ↑ Serum protein ↓ Serum albumin ↓	Heavy proteinuria >5 g/day
Pyelonephritis	Cloudy Protein Nitrite Leukocytes	WBCs WBC casts Bacteria RBCs	Positive ACB test	Concentrating ability decreased in chronic cases

prognosis, progressing to chronic renal failure within 10 years. The laboratory findings are variable; however, hematuria, proteinuria, and decreased serum complement levels are frequent findings.

Focal Glomerulonephritis

In contrast to other forms of glomerulonephritis, focal glomerulonephritis affects only a certain number of glomeruli, whereas the others remain normal.[15] Symptoms are often similar to other glomerular diseases, including the nephrotic syndrome and minimal change disease. Immune deposits are a frequent finding and are often seen in undamaged glomeruli. Microscopic and macroscopic hematuria and proteinuria are routine laboratory findings.

Minimal Change Disease

As the name implies, minimal change disease produces little cellular change in the glomerulus. Patients are frequently children who present with edema, heavy proteinuria, lipiduria, and transient hematuria. Although the etiology is unknown at this time, allergic reactions, recent immunizations, and possession of the HLA-B12 antigen have been associated. The prognosis is generally good, with frequent complete remissions.

RENAL FAILURE

Acute renal failure as a result of acute tubular necrosis may result from renal vasoconstriction or direct tubular damage from nephrotoxic agents. Hypotension caused by traumatic or surgical shock, burns, and intravascular hemolysis, as occurs in transfusion reactions, are frequent causes of acute renal failure. Chronic renal failure is not an uncommon complication of the forms of glomerulonephritis discussed previously. Laboratory findings include decreased glomerular filtration rate, lack of renal concentrating ability, and increased serum BUN and creatinine. Routine urinalysis results will reflect the cause of the renal failure.

PYELONEPHRITIS

Acute pyelonephritis is most frequently seen in women, often resulting from untreated cases of cystitis or lower urinary tract infection, and does not cause permanent damage to the renal tubules. Recurrent infections caused by structural abnormalities or obstructions of the urinary tract allow bacteria to remain in the kidney, resulting in tubular damage and chronic pyelonephritis.[20]

Urinalysis findings in both acute and chronic pyelonephritis are similar and include white blood cells—often in clumps—white blood cell casts, bacteria, positive nitrite reactions, and possible proteinuria and hematuria. With the exception of the presence of white blood cell casts that are indicative of tubular involvement, similar results will be found with infections of the lower urinary tract such as cystitis. Differentiation using the immunofluorescent antibody-coated bacteria (ACB) test may be necessary. Bacteria exposed to the antibody-rich inflamed tissue of the renal tubules are more likely to produce a positive ACB test.[18]

REFERENCES

1. Assadi, F and Fornell, L: Estimation of urine specific gravity in neonates with a reagent strip. J Pediatr 108(6):995–996, 1986.
2. Bartter, F and Delea, C: Diabetes insipidus: Its nature and diagnosis. Lab Man 20(1):23–28, 1982.
3. Bauer, JD: Clinical Laboratory Methods. CV Mosby, St Louis, 1982.
4. Benitez, O, et al: Inaccuracy in neonatal measurement of urine concentration with a refractometer. J Pediatr 108(4):613–616, 1986.
5. Bianchi, C: Noninvasive methods for the measurement of renal function. In Duart,

C (ed): Renal Function Tests: Clinical Laboratory Procedures and Diagnosis. Little, Brown & Co, Boston, 1980.

6. Campbell, J and Campbell, JB: Laboratory Mathematics. CV Mosby, St Louis, 1980.

7. Chachati, A, et al: Rapid method for the measurement of differential renal function: Validation. J Nucl Med 28(5):829–836, 1987.

8. Chan, J: Renal acidosis. In Duart, C (ed): Renal Function Tests: Clinical Laboratory Procedures and Diagnosis. Little, Brown & Co, Boston, 1980.

9. Draviam, EJ, Custer, EM, and Schoen, I: Vapor pressure and freezing point osmolality measurements applied to a volatile screen. Am J Clin Pathol 82(6):706–709, 1984.

10. Duston, H and Corcoran, A: Functional interpretation of renal tests. Med Clin North Am 39:947–956, 1955.

11. Forland, M (ed): Nephrology. Medical Examination Publishing, New York, 1983.

12. Gabriel, R: Time to scrap creatinine clearance? Br Med J 13(293):1568, 1986.

13. Glassock, RJ, et al: Primary glomerular diseases. In Brenner, BM and Rector, FC: The Kidney. WB Saunders, Philadelphia, 1986.

14. Heptinstall, RH: Pathology of the Kidney, Vol 1. Little, Brown & Co, Boston, 1983.

15. Heptinstall, RH: Pathology of the Kidney, Vol 2. Little, Brown & Co, Boston, 1983.

16. Heptinstall, RH: Pathology of the Kidney, Vol 3. Little, Brown & Co, Boston, 1983.

17. Jacobsen, FK, et al: Evaluation of kidney function after meals. Lancet i(8163): 319–320, 1980.

18. Jennette, JC: The pathophysiologic effects of infections on the kidneys. J Med Tech 4(4):165–170, 1987.

19. Juel, R: Serum osmolality: A CAP survey analysis. Am J Clin Pathol 68:165–167, 1977.

20. Kurtz, SB: Urinary tract infections. In Knox, FG (ed): Textbook of Renal Pathophysiology. JB Lippincott, Philadelphia, 1978.

21. Mercier, DE, Feld, RD, and Witte, DI: Comparison of dewpoint and freezing point osmometry. Am J Med Technol 44(11):1066–1069, 1978.

22. Murphy, JE, Preuss, HG, and Henry, JB: Evaluation of renal function and water, electrolyte and acid-base balance. In Henry, JB (ed): Clinical Diagnosis and Management by Laboratory Methods. WB Saunders, Philadelphia, 1984.

23. Murray, B and Ferris, TF: Blood and urinary chemistries in the evaluation of renal function. Semin Nephrol 5(3):208–221, 1985.

24. Oken, D: Osmometry and differential diagnosis. In Lauler, D (ed): Urinalysis in the 70's. Medcom, New York, 1973.

25. Payne, RB: Creatinine clearance: A redundant clinical investigation. Annals Clin Biochem 23:243–250, 1986.

26. Peterson, L: β_2 Microglobulin. Clin Chem News 14(1):6, 1988.

27. Price, JD and Durnford, J: Laboratory test for kidney function: Urea or creatinine? Lancet i(8140):420–422, 1979.

28. Schoeff, L: Antidiuretic hormone and water regulation. J Med Technol 3(6):342–346, 1986.

29. Schnurr, E, Lahme, W, and Kuppers, H: Measurement of renal clearance of inulin and PAH in the steady state without urine collection. Clin Nephrol 13(1):26–29, 1980.

30. Vader, A: Renal Physiology. McGraw-Hill, New York, 1980.

31. Weisberg, HF: Osmolality. Lab Med 12(2):81–85, 1981.

STUDY QUESTIONS (Choose one best answer)

1. Each kidney is composed of approximately
   a. 100 nephrons
   b. 1,000 nephrons
   c. 10,000 nephrons
   d. 1,000,000 nephrons

2. The total renal blood flow is approximately
   a. 60 ml/min
   b. 120 ml/min
   c. 600 ml/min
   d. 1200 ml/min

3. The normal kidney performs all of the following functions except
   a. removes metabolic waste products from the blood
   b. regulates the acid-base balance in the body
   c. removes excess protein from the blood
   d. regulates the water content in the body

4. The glomerular filtrate is described as
   a. a protein filtrate of plasma
   b. a glucose- and protein-containing filtrate of plasma
   c. a plasma filtrate without glucose and protein
   d. an ultrafiltrate of plasma that does not contain protein

5. The specific gravity of the fluid leaving the glomerulus is
   a. 1.001
   b. 1.010
   c. 1.020
   d. 1.030

6. In the proximal convoluted tubule, glucose is reabsorbed by active transport, and urea, by passive transport. For active transport to occur,
   a. glucose must combine with a carrier protein, creating electrochemical energy
   b. glucose must be filtered through the tubular membranes
   c. glucose concentration in the tubular filtrate must be higher than in the blood
   d. glucose concentration in the blood must be higher than in the tubular filtrate

7. The renal threshold for glucose is
   a. 50–100 mg/dl
   b. 160–180 mg/dl
   c. 220–240 mg/dl
   d. over 240 mg/dl

8. Concentration of the tubular filtrate by the countercurrent mechanism is dependent on all of the following except
   a. high salt concentration in the renal medulla
   b. water-impermeable walls in the ascending loop of Henle
   c. reabsorption of sodium and chloride in the ascending loop of Henle
   d. active transport of glucose and amino acids in the proximal convoluted tubule

9. Aldosterone and ADH are
   a. hormones that regulate the reabsorption of glucose
   b. hormones that regulate the permeability of the tubular walls in the descending and ascending loops of Henle
   c. hormones that regulate the countercurrent mechanism
   d. hormones that regulate final urine volume and sodium content

10. The majority of the filtered sodium is reabsorbed in the

    a. proximal convoluted tubule
    b. descending loop of Henle
    c. ascending loop of Henle
    d. distal convoluted tubule

11. Substances removed from the blood by tubular secretion include primarily

    a. protein, hydrogen, and ammonia
    b. protein, hydrogen, and potassium
    c. protein-bound substances, hydrogen, and potassium
    d. amino acids, hydrogen, and ammonia

12. Clearance tests for glomerular filtration must use substances that are

    a. not filtered by the glomerulus
    b. completely reabsorbed in the proximal convoluted tubule
    c. secreted in the distal convoluted tubule
    d. neither reabsorbed nor secreted by the tubules

13. The most common cause of error in the creatinine clearance test is

    a. miscalculation of chemical results
    b. variation in serum creatinine levels
    c. improperly collected urine specimens
    d. diet high in vegetables

14. A clearance test is reported as

    a. milligrams per deciliter
    b. milligrams per 24 hours
    c. milliliters per 24 hours
    d. milliliters per minute

15. Calculate the creatinine clearance of a 6-hour specimen using the following data:

    urine creatinine   = 90 mg/dl
    plasma creatinine = 1.8 mg/dl
    urine volume   = 720 ml

16. A 6-year old child has a total body surface of 0.86 square meters. Calculate the creatinine clearance from a 4-hour specimen with a volume of 120 ml, urine creatinine of 150 mg/dl, and plasma creatinine of 1.5 mg/dl.

17. John White donates one of his two healthy kidneys to his twin brother. His glomerular filtration rate can be expected to

    a. decrease by 50 percent
    b. increase by 50 percent
    c. decrease gradually over 1 year
    d. remain essentially unchanged

18. One of the three morning specimens collected in a Fishberg concentration test should have a specific gravity of at least

    a. 1.002
    b. 1.010
    c. 1.022
    d. 1.034

19. Lack of tubular concentrating ability is indicated when the Mosenthal test shows

    a. high specific gravity and low volume in the night specimen
    b. low specific gravity and high volume in the night specimen
    c. specific gravity over 1.026 in the day specimen
    d. specific gravity over 1.010 and volume over 300 ml in the night specimen

20. An osmole is defined as
    a. 1 gram molecular weight of a substance
    b. 1 gram equivalent weight of a substance
    c. 1 gram molecular weight of a substance divided by the number of its dissociation particles
    d. 1 gram equivalent weight of a substance divided by the number of its dissociation particles

21. Measurement of urine osmolarity is a more accurate measure of renal concentrating ability than specific gravity measured by urinometer because
    a. osmolarity is measured by instrumentation
    b. specific gravity is not influenced by urea and glucose molecules
    c. specific gravity measures only urea and glucose concentrations
    d. osmolarity is influenced equally by large and small molecules

22. Osmometers utilizing the freezing point colligative property of solutions are based on the principle that
    a. 1 osmole of nonionizing substance dissolved in 1 kilogram of water raises the freezing point 1.86°C
    b. 1 osmole of nonionizing substance dissolved in 1 kilogram of water lowers the freezing point 1.86°C
    c. increased solute concentration will raise the freezing point of water in direct proportion to an NaCl standard
    d. decreased solute concentration will decrease the freezing point in direct proportion to an NaCl standard

23. Vapor pressure osmometers are based on the principle that
    a. increased solute raises the vapor pressure of a solution
    b. increased solute lowers the vapor pressure of a solution
    c. increased solute raises the dew-point temperature of a solution
    d. a and c but not b are correct

24. Substances that may interfere with the measurement of urine and serum osmolarity include all of the following except
    a. ethanol
    b. lactic acid
    c. sodium
    d. lipids

25. The normal serum osmolarity is
    a. 50–100 mOsm
    b. 275–300 mOsm
    c. 400–500 mOsm
    d. 3 times the urine osmolarity

26. A free water clearance of +3.0 could be indicative of
    a. dehydration
    b. lack of renal concentration and dilution
    c. diabetes insipidus
    d. increased ADH production

27. The PSP test can be used as a measure of
    a. renal concentration
    b. renal secretion
    c. renal urine flow
    d. glomerular filtration

28. The most informative specimen in the PSP test is the

    a. 15–minute specimen
    b. 30–minute specimen
    c. 1–hour specimen
    d. 2–hour specimen

29. To provide an accurate measure of renal blood flow, a test substance should be

    a. completely filtered by the glomerulus
    b. completely reabsorbed by the tubules
    c. completely secreted when it reaches the distal convoluted tubule
    d. completely cleared on each contact with functional renal tissue

30. A steady infusion of p-aminohippuric acid is given to a patient over a 1–hour pe-
    riod, and 90 ml of urine are collected during this time. Calculate the patient's renal
    blood flow using a urine PAH concentration of 360 mg/dl and a plasma PAH con-
    centration of 0.8 mg/dl.

31. Renal tubular acidosis can be caused by

    a. the production of excessively acidic urine due to increased filtration of hydrogen
       ions
    b. the production of excessively acidic urine due to increased secretion of hydrogen
       ions
    c. the inability to produce an acidic urine due to impaired production of ammonia
    d. the inability to produce an acidic urine due to the increased production of
       ammonia

32. Match the following routine urinalysis results with the most probable renal function
    abnormality:

    _____ 2+ protein   a. decreased ammonia production
    _____ 4+ glucose   b. oliguria
    _____ 1.002 specific gravity   c. proximal convoluted tubule damage
    _____ pH 8.0   d. increased ADH
    _____ broad casts   e. glomerular membrane damage
                                        f. decreased ADH
                                        g. increased renal blood flow

3

Physical Examination of the Urine

LEARNING OBJECTIVES

Upon completion of this chapter, readers will be able to

1. list the common terminology used to report normal urine color.
2. discuss the relationship of urochrome to normal urine color.
3. tell how the presence of bilirubin in a specimen may be suspected.
4. discuss the significance of cloudy red urine and clear red urine.
5. name two pathologic causes of black or brown urine.
6. discuss the significance of Pyridium in a specimen.
7. define appearance.
8. list the common terminology used to report appearance.
9. describe the appearance and discuss the significance of amorphous phosphates and amorphous urates in freshly voided urine.
10. list three pathologic and four nonpathologic causes of cloudy urine.
11. define specific gravity and tell why this measurement can be significant in the routine analysis.
12. describe the principles of physics used in measuring specific gravity by urinometer and refractometer.
13. given the calibration temperature and specimen temperature, calculate a temperature correction for a specific gravity reading determined by urinometer.
14. given the concentration of glucose and protein in a specimen, calculate the correction needed to compensate for these high molecular-weight substances in the urinometer specific gravity reading.
15. name two nonpathogenic causes of abnormally high specific gravity readings.

As mentioned in chapter 1, early physicians based many medical decisions on the color and appearance of urine. Today, observation of these characteristics provides preliminary information concerning disorders such as glomerular bleeding, liver disease, inborn errors of metabolism, and urinary tract infection. Measurement of specific gravity aids in the evaluation of renal tubular function. The results of the physical portion of the urinalysis can also be used to confirm or to explain findings in the chemical and microscopic areas of the urinalysis.

COLOR

The color of urine varies from almost colorless to black. These variations may be due to normal metabolic functions, physical activity, ingested materials, or pathologic conditions. A noticeable change in urine color is often the reason a patient seeks medical advice, and it then becomes the responsibility of the laboratory to determine whether this color change is normal or pathologic.

NORMAL URINE COLOR

Terminology used to describe the color of normal urine may differ slightly among laboratories. Common descriptions include pale yellow, straw, light yellow, yellow, dark yellow, and amber. Care should be taken to examine the specimen under a good light source, looking down through the container against a white background. The yellow color of urine is due to the presence of a pigment, which was named urochrome by Thudichum in 1864. Urochrome is a product of endogenous metabolism, and under normal conditions it is produced at a constant rate. The actual amount of urochrome produced is dependent on the body's metabolic state, with increased amounts being produced in thyroid conditions and fasting states.[4] Urochrome also increases in urine that stands at room temperature.[10]

Because urochrome is excreted at a constant rate, the intensity of the yellow color in a fresh urine specimen can give a rough estimate of urine concentration. A dilute urine will be pale yellow, and a concentrated specimen will be dark yellow. Remember that, due to variations in the body's state of hydration, these differences in the yellow color of urine are normal.

ABNORMAL URINE COLOR

Dark yellow or amber urine may not always signify a normal concentrated urine but can be caused by the presence of the abnormal pigment bilirubin. If bilirubin is present, it will be detected during the chemical examination; however, its presence is suspected if a yellow foam appears when the specimen is shaken. A urine specimen that contains bilirubin may also contain hepatitis virus.

As can be seen in Table 3–1, abnormal urine colors are as numerous as their causes; however, certain colors are seen more frequently and have a greater clinical significance than others. One of the most common causes of abnormal urine color is the presence of blood. Red is the usual color imparted to urine by blood, but the color may range from pink to black, depending on the amount of blood, the pH of the urine, and the length of contact. Red blood cells remaining in an acidic urine for several hours will produce a brown-black urine due to the denaturation of hemoglobin. A fresh brown-black urine containing red blood cells may also be indicative of glomerular bleeding.[1] Besides red blood cells, two other substances, hemoglobin and myoglobin, produce a red urine and result in a positive chemical test for blood. When red blood cells are present, the urine will be red and cloudy; however, if hemoglobin or myoglobin is present, the specimen is red and clear. It may be possible to distinguish between hemoglobinuria and myoglobinuria by examining the patient's plasma. Hemoglobinuria resulting from the in-vivo breakdown of red blood cells is accompanied by red plasma; whereas myoglobinuria is produced by skeletal muscle and does not affect the color of the plasma. The possibility of hemoglobinuria being produced from the in-vitro lysis of red blood cells must also be considered. Chemical tests to distinguish between hemoglobin and myoglobin are available (see chapter 4). Additional testing is also recommended for urine specimens that turn brown or black upon standing and have negative chemical tests for blood, inasmuch as they may contain melanin or homogentisic acid (see chapter 6).

Many abnormal urine colors are of a nonpathogenic nature and are caused by the ingestion of highly pigmented foods, medications, and vitamins. Eating fresh beets will produce a red urine in certain genetically susceptible persons, and chewing Clorets can result in green urine.[5, 11]

Observation of specimen collection bags from hospitalized patients frequently detects abnormally colored urine. This may signify a pathologic condition that requires the urine to stand for a period of time before color development, or it may be due to medica-

TABLE 3–1. Laboratory Correlation of Urine Color[3]

COLOR	CAUSE	LABORATORY CORRELATIONS
Colorless Straw Pale yellow	Recent fluid consumption	Commonly observed with random specimens
	Polyuria or diabetes insipidus	Increased 24-hour volume
	Diabetes mellitus	Elevated specific gravity and positive glucose test
Dark yellow Amber Orange	Concentrated specimen	May be normal after strenuous exercise or in a first morning specimen
		Dehydration from fever or burns
	Bilirubin	Yellow foam when shaken and positive chemical tests for bilirubin
	Acriflavine	Negative bile tests and possible green fluorescence
	Carrots or vitamin A	Soluble in petroleum ether
	Pyridium	Drug commonly administered for urinary tract infections
		May have orange foam and thick orange pigment that can obscure or interfere with dipstick readings
	Nitrofurantoin	Antibiotic administered for urinary tract infections
Yellow-green Yellow-brown	Bilirubin oxidized to biliverdin	Colored foam in acidic urine, and false- negative chemical tests for bilirubin
	Rhubarb	Seen in acidic urine
Green Blue-green	*Pseudomonas* infection	Positive urine culture
	Amitriptyline	Antidepressant
	Methocarbamol	Muscle relaxant
	Clorets	None
	Indican	Confirm with Obermayer's test
	Methylene blue	None
	Phenol	When oxidized
Pink Red	Red blood cells	Cloudy urine with positive chemical tests for blood and RBCs visible microscopically
	Hemoglobin	Clear urine with positive chemical tests for blood; plasma may be red
	Myoglobin	Clear urine with positive chemical tests for blood; plasma will be colorless
		Specific identification tests available
	Porphyrins	Negative chemical tests for blood
		Detect with Watson-Schwartz screening test or fluorescence under ultraviolet light
	Beets	Alkaline urine of genetically susceptible persons
	Phenolsulfonphthalein	Alkaline urines after PSP test for renal function
	Bromsulphalein	Alkaline urines after BSP test for liver function
	Rhubarb	Seen in alkaline urine
	Menstrual contamination	Cloudy specimen with red blood cells, mucus, and clots
	Phenindione	Anticoagulant

TABLE 3–1. *Continued*

COLOR	CAUSE	LABORATORY CORRELATIONS
Brown Black	Red blood cells oxidized to methemoglobin	Seen in acidic urine after standing; positive chemical test for blood
	Myoglobin	Positive chemical test for blood
	Homogentisic acid (Alkaptonuria)	Seen in alkaline urine after standing; specific tests are available
	Melanin or melanogen	Urine darkens upon standing and reacts with nitroprusside and ferric chloride
	Phenol derivatives	Interferes with copper reduction tests
	Argyrol (antiseptic)	Color disappears with ferric chloride
	Methyldopa or levodopa	Antihypertensive
	Metronidazole	Flagyl, darkens on standing

tions. Phenol derivatives found in certain intravenous medications will produce green urine upon oxidation.[2] Medications and bacteria may also react with the material of the specimen bag to produce the abnormal color.[12]

Also frequently encountered in the urinalysis laboratory is the yellow-orange specimen caused by the administration of Pyridium compounds to persons with urinary tract infections. This thick, orange pigment not only obscures the natural color of the specimen but also interferes with chemical tests based on color reactions. Recognition of the presence of Pyridium in a specimen is important so that alternate testing procedures can be used.

APPEARANCE

Appearance is a general term that refers to the clarity of a urine specimen. In a routine urinalysis, appearance is determined in the same manner used by the ancient physicians, that is, by visually examining the mixed specimen while holding it in front of a light source. The specimen should, of course, be in a clear container. Inasmuch as many disposable plastic containers are made of nontransparent plastic, it may be necessary to transfer the specimen. Pouring the specimen into a centrifuge tube and examining it prior to centrifugation can be a time-saving step. Common terminology used to report appearance includes clear, hazy, slightly cloudy, cloudy, turbid, and milky.

NORMAL APPEARANCE

Freshly voided normal urine is usually clear; however, cloudiness caused by the precipitation of amorphous phosphates and carbonates usually appears as white clouds in the specimen. Normal acidic urine may also appear cloudy because of precipitated amorphous urates, calcium oxalate, or uric acid crystals. The cloudiness in acidic urine often resembles brick dust owing to the accumulation of the pink pigment uroerythrin on the surface of the crystals. Uroerythrin is a normal constituent of urine. The presence of squamous epithelial cells and mucus, particularly in specimens from women, will also result in a hazy but normal urine.

TURBIDITY

Besides amorphous crystals, the four most common substances that cause turbidity in urine are white blood cells, red blood cells, epithelial cells, and bacteria.[13] Other causes

TABLE 3–2. Laboratory Correlations in Urine Turbidity[3]

ACIDIC URINE
   Amorphous urates
   X-ray contrast media

ALKALINE URINE
   Amorphous phosphates, carbonates

SOLUBLE WITH HEAT
   Amorphous urates, uric acid crystals

SOLUBLE IN DILUTE ACETIC ACID
   Red blood cells
   Amorphous phosphates, carbonates

INSOLUBLE IN DILUTE ACETIC ACID
   White blood cells
   Bacteria, yeast
   Spermatozoa

SOLUBLE IN ETHER
   Lipids
   Lymphatic fluid, chyle

of turdibity include lipids, semen, mucus, lymph fluid, crystals, yeast, fecal material, and extraneous contamination, such as talcum powder and x-ray contrast media. Many of these substances are nonpathogenic. However, because as white blood cells, red blood cells, and bacteria are indicative of pathogenicity, a fresh, turbid specimen can be a cause for concern. The clarity of a urine specimen certainly provides a key to the microscopic examination results, because the degree of turbidity should correspond with the amount of material observed under the microscope. Questionable causes of urine turbidity can be confirmed by the simple chemical tests shown in Table 3–2.

It must also be kept in mind that a clear urine is not always normal. However, with the increased sensitivity of the routine chemical tests, which include a chemical test for leukocytes, most abnormalities in clear urine will be detected prior to the microscopic analysis. It has even been suggested that by accurately measuring turbidity by means of nephelometry, it may be possible to omit the microscopic examination on routine specimens with no degree of turbidity.[13]

SPECIFIC GRAVITY

The kidney's ability to selectively reabsorb essential chemicals and water from the glomerular filtrate is one of the body's most important functions. The intricate process of reabsorption is often the first renal function to become impaired; therefore, an assessment of the kidney's ability to reabsorb is a necessary component of the routine urinalysis. This evaluation is accomplished by measuring the specific gravity of the specimen. Specific gravity also will detect possible dehydration or abnormalities in antidiuretic hormone (ADH) and can be used to determine whether specimen concentration is adequate to ensure accuracy of chemical tests.[6, 7]

Specific gravity is defined as the density of a substance compared with the density of a similar volume of distilled water at a similar temperature. Because urine is actually water that contains dissolved chemicals, the specific gravity of urine is a measure of the density of the dissolved chemicals in the specimen. Because it is a measure of specimen density, specific gravity is influenced not only by the number of particles present but also by their size. Large urea molecules contribute more to the reading than do the small sodium and chloride molecules. Therefore, as urea is of less value than sodium and chloride in the evaluation of renal concentrating ability, it also may be necessary to test the specimen's osmolarity. This procedure is discussed in chapter 2. However, for purposes of routine urinalysis, the specific gravity provides valuable preliminary information and can be easily performed using either a urinometer (hydrometer), a refractometer, or reagent strip.

URINOMETER

The urinometer consists of a weighted float attached to a scale that has been calibrated in terms of urine specific gravity (1.000 to 1.040). The weighted float displaces a volume of liquid equal to its weight and has been designed to sink to a level of 1.000 in distilled water. The additional mass provided by the dissolved substances in urine causes the float to displace a volume of urine smaller than that of distilled water. The level to which the urinometer sinks, as shown in Figure 3–1, is representative of the specimen's mass or specific gravity.

The major disadvantage of using a urinometer to measure specific gravity is that it requires a large volume (10 to 15 ml) of specimen. The container in which the urinometer is floated must be wide enough to allow it to float without touching the sides, and the volume of urine must be sufficient to prevent the urinometer from resting on the bottom. When using the urinometer, an adequate amount of urine is first poured into a proper-size container, and the urinometer is then added with a spinning motion. The scale reading is then taken at the bottom of the urine meniscus.

It may also be necessary to correct the urinometer reading for temperature, inasmuch as urinometers are calibrated to read 1.000 in distilled water at a particular temperature. The calibration temperature is printed on the instrument and is usually about 20°C. If the specimen is cold, 0.001 must be subtracted from the reading for every 3 degrees that the specimen temperature is below the urinometer calibration temperature. Conversely, 0.001 must be added to the reading for every 3 degrees that the specimen measures above the calibration temperature.

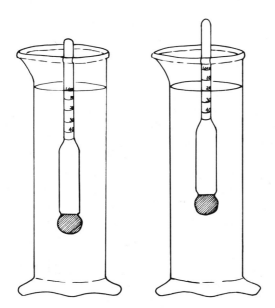

FIGURE 3–1. Urinometers representing various specific gravity readings.

Example: A refrigerated specimen with a temperature of 14°C gives a specific gravity reading of 1.020. Calculate the correct reading.

20° (calibration temperature) − 14° = 6°

$$\frac{6°}{3°} \times 0.001 = 0.002$$

1.020 − 0.002 = 1.018 corrected specific gravity

Temperature corrections are not necessary when specific gravity is determined using a refractometer, because readings are automatically corrected for temperature.

A correction must also be calculated when using either the urinometer or the refractometer if large amounts of glucose or protein are present. Both glucose and protein are high-molecular-weight substances that have no relationship to renal concentrating ability but will increase specimen density. Therefore, their contribution to the specific gravity is subtracted to give a more accurate report of the kidney's concentrating ability. A gram of protein per deciliter of urine will raise the urine specific gravity by 0.003, and a gram of glucose per deciliter will add 0.004 to the reading. Consequently, for each gram of protein present, 0.003 must be subtracted from the specific gravity reading, and 0.004 must be subtracted for each gram of glucose present.

Example: A. A specimen containing 1 gram of protein and 1 gram of glucose per deciliter has a specific gravity reading of 1.030. Calculate the corrected reading.

1.030 − 0.003 (protein) = 1.027 − 0.004 (glucose)

= 1.023 corrected specific gravity

B. A refrigerated specimen has a temperature of 17°C and contains 2 grams of protein per deciliter. The urinometer reading is 1.032. Calculate the corrected reading.

20°C − 17°C = 3°C = 0.001 (temperature correction)

$$0.003 \times 2\ g = \frac{0.006}{0.007}\ \text{(protein correction)}$$

1.032 − 0.007 = 1.025

REFRACTOMETER

The refractometer, like the urinometer, determines the concentration of dissolved particles in a specimen. It does this by measuring refractive index. Refractive index is a comparison of the velocity of light in air with the velocity of light in a solution. The velocity is dependent on the concentration of dissolved particles present in the solution and determines the angle at which light passes through a solution. The clinical refractometer (TS Meter, AO Scientific Instruments Division, Buffalo, NY) makes use of these principles of light by measuring the angle at which light passing through a solution enters a prism and mathematically converts this angle (refractive index) to specific gravity.

The refractometer provides the distinct advantage of determining specific gravity using a small volume of specimen (1 or 2 drops). Temperature corrections are not necessary because the instrument is temperature compensated between 60°F and 100°F. Corrections for glucose and protein are still calculated, although refractometer readings are less affected by particle density than are urinometer readings.[8] When using the refractometer, a drop of urine is placed on the prism, the instrument is focused at a good light source, and the reading is taken directly from the specific gravity scale (Fig. 3–2). The prism and its cover should be cleaned after each specimen is tested.

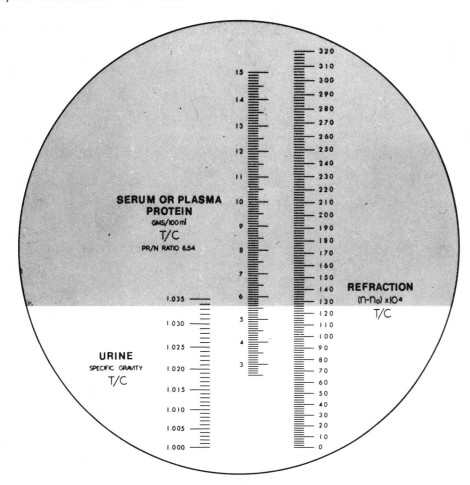

FIGURE 3–2. Refractometer scale. (From Instructions for Use and Care of the AO TS Meter. Warner Lambert Technologies, Buffalo, NY, with permission. Courtesy of Reichert Scientific Instruments.)

Calibration of the refractometer is performed using distilled water that should read 1.000. If necessary, the instrument contains a 0 set screw to adjust the distilled water reading. The calibration is further checked using 5 percent NaCl, which must read 1.022 ± 0.001, or 9 percent sucrose that should read 1.034 ± 0.001. Control samples representing low, medium, and high concentrations should also be run at the beginning of each shift. Calibration and control results are always recorded in the appropriate quality control records. A semiautomated instrument (Digital Urinometer, Biovation, Inc., Richmond, CA) that employs the principle of refractive index is also available. Specimens are poured across the prism, and readings are displayed on a digital readout screen.

In addition to using the urinometer and refractometer, specific gravity can be determined chemically by dipstick (see chapter 4) and by the falling drop method. The automated urinalysis instrument (Clinilab, Ames Company, Elkhart, IN) uses a falling drop method to measure specific gravity. The instrument determines the amount of time it takes a drop of urine to fall a fixed distance through an insolvent liquid and converts this time to specific gravity.

CLINICAL CORRELATIONS

The specific gravity of the plasma filtrate entering the glomerulus is 1.010. The term isosthenuric is used to describe urine with a specific gravity of 1.010. Specimens below

1.010 are hyposthenuric, and those above 1.010 are hypersthenuric. One would expect urine that has been concentrated by the kidney to be hypersthenuric; however, this is not always true. Normal random specimens may range from 1.001 to 1.035, depending on the patient's degree of hydration. The majority of random specimens fall between 1.015 and 1.025, and any random specimen with a specific gravity of 1.023 or higher is generally considered normal. If a patient exhibits consistently low results, procedures are available for collecting specimens under conditions of controlled fluid intake (see chapter 2).

Abnormally high results—over 1.035—are seen in patients who have recently undergone an intravenous pyelogram. This is caused by the excretion of the injected x-ray contrast media. Patients who are receiving dextran or other high-molecular-weight intravenous fluids will also produce urine with an abnormally high specific gravity. Once the foreign substance has been cleared from the body, the specific gravity will return to normal. In these circumstances, urine concentration can be measured using the reagent strip chemical test or osmometry.[14] When the presence of glucose or protein is the cause of high results, this will be detected in the routine chemical examination. As discussed earlier, this can be corrected for mathematically. Should it become necessary to determine the true specific gravity of a previously diluted specimen, the decimal portion of the observed specific gravity is multiplied by the dilution factor. A specimen diluted 1:2 with a reading of 1.010 would have an actual specific gravity of 1.020.

ODOR

Although it is seldom of clinical significance and is not a part of the routine urinalysis, urine odor is a noticeable physical property. Freshly voided urine has a faint odor of aromatic compounds. As the specimen stands, the odor of ammonia becomes predominant. The breakdown of urea is responsible for the characteristic ammonia odor. Causes of unusual odors include bacterial infections, which cause a strong, unpleasant odor, and diabetic ketones, which cause a sweet or fruity odor. A serious metabolic defect results in urine with a strong odor of maple syrup and is appropriately called maple syrup urine disease (see chapter 6). Ingestion of certain foods, particularly asparagus, can cause an unusual or pungent urine odor. Studies have shown that although everyone who eats asparagus produces an odor, only certain genetically predisposed people can smell the odor.[9]

REFERENCES

1. Berman, L: When urine is red. JAMA 237:2753–2754, 1977.
2. Bowling, P, Belliveau, RR, and Butler,TJ: Intravenous medications and green urine. JAMA 246(3):216, 1981.
3. Bradley, M and Schumann, BB: Examination of the urine. In Henry, JB (ed): Clinical Diagnosis and Management by Laboratory Methods. WB Saunders, Philadelphia, 1984, pp 380–458.
4. Drabkin, DL: The normal pigment of urine: The relationship of urinary pigment output to diet and metabolism. J Biol Chem 75:443–479, 1927.
5. Evans, B: The greening of urine: Still another "Cloret sign." N Engl J Med 300(4):202, 1979.
6. Free, AH: A Colourimetric method for urine specific gravity compared with current direct and indirect procedures. Br J Clin Pract 36(9):307–311, 1982.
7. Kavelman, DA: A representative of Ames responds. Clin Chem 29(1):210–211, 1983.
8. Low, PS and Tay, JSH: Urine: Osmolality refractive index and specific gravity. J Singapore Paediatr Soc 20(1):37–42, 1978.

9. Mitchell, SC et al: Odorous urine following asparagus ingestion in man. Experienta 43(4):382–383, 1987.

10. Ostow, M and Philo, S: The chief urinary pigment: The relationship between the rate of excretion of the yellow pigment and the metabolic rate. Am J Med Sci 207:507–512, 1944.

11. Reimann, HA: Re: Red urine. JAMA 241(22):2380, 1979.

12. Rovers, J et al: Apparent urine discoloration from drainage bag stain. Drug Intell Clin Pharm 21(3):295,1987.

STUDY QUESTIONS (Choose one best answer)

1. The normal yellow color of urine is produced by
   a. bilirubin
   b. urobilinogen
   c. urochrome
   d. hemoglobin

2. A yellow-brown specimen that produces a yellow foam when shaken can be suspected of containing
   a. bilirubin
   b. hemoglobin
   c. carrots
   d. rhubarb

3. All of the following can contribute to the color of a urine specimen that contains blood except
   a. amount of blood
   b. type of specimen
   c. pH of specirnen
   d. length of contact

4. Specimens that contain intact red blood cells can be visually distinguished from those that contain hemoglobin because
   a. hemoglobin produces a much brighter red color
   b. hemoglobin produces a cloudy, pink specimen
   c. red blood cells produce a cloudy specimen
   d. red blood cells are quickly converted to hemoglobin

5. After eating beets purchased at the local farmers' market, Mrs. Williams notices that her urine is red, but Mr. Williams's urine remains yellow. The Williamses should
   a. be concerned because red urine always indicates the presence of blood
   b. not be concerned because all women produce red urine after eating beets
   c. be concerned because both of them should have red urine if beets are the cause
   d. not be concerned because only Mrs. Williams is genetically susceptible to producing red urine from beets

6. Specimens from patients receiving treatment for urinary tract infections frequently appear
   a. clear and red
   b. thick and orange
   c. dilute and pale yellow
   d. cloudy and red

7. Freshly voided normal urine is usually clear; however, if it is alkaline, a white turbidity may be present due to

   a. amorphous phosphates and carbonates
   b. white blood cells
   c. uroerythrin
   d. yeast

8. Turbidity in normal acidic urine

   a. is never observed
   b. is caused by disintegrated epithelial cells
   c. resembles brick dust due to uroerythrin on crystals
   d. resembles a granular white precipitate

9. Which of the following specific gravities would be most likely to correlate with a pale yellow urine?

   a. 1.005
   b. 1.015
   c. 1.025
   d. 1.035

10. Specific gravity is a measure of

    a. particle content
    b. molecular weight
    c. molarity
    d. density

11. Calculate the corrected specific gravity using the following data:

urinometer reading	= 1.025
urine temperature	= 14°C
urinometer calibration temperature	= 20°C
urine glucose	= 2.0 g/dl
urine protein	= 2000 mg/dl

12. A urine specific gravity measured by refractometer is 1.029, and the temperature of the urine is 14°C. The specific gravity should be reported as

    a. 1.019
    b. 1.026
    c. 1.029
    d. 1.032

13. Refractive index compares

    a. light velocity in solutions with light velocity in solids
    b. light velocity in air with light velocity in solutions
    c. light scattering by air with light scattering by solutions
    d. light scattering by particles in solution

14. Refractometers are calibrated using

    a. distilled water and protein
    b. distilled water and blood
    c. distilled water and sodium chloride
    d. distilled water and urea

15. A correlation exists between a specific gravity of 1.050 and a

    a. 2+ glucose
    b. 2+ protein
    c. first morning specimen
    d. radiographic dye infusion

16. An alkaline urine turns black upon standing, develops a cloudy white precipitate, and has a specific gravity of 1.002. The major concern about this specimen would be

    a. color
    b. turbidity
    c. specific gravity
    d. all of the above

17. The reading of distilled water of the refractometer is 1.003. You should

    a. subtract 1.003 from each specimen reading
    b. add 1.003 to each specimen reading
    c. use a new refractometer
    d. adjust the set screw

18. A urine specimen with a specific gravity of 1.005 has been diluted 1:10. The actual specific gravity is

    a. 1.005
    b. 1.050
    c. 1.055
    d. 10.050

CHEMICAL EXAMINATION OF THE URINE

LEARNING OBJECTIVES

Upon completion of this chapter, readers will be able to

1. describe the proper technique for performing chemical tests on urine by reagent strip and give possible errors if this technique is not followed.
2. list four causes of premature deterioration of reagent strips and tell how to avoid them.
3. list five quality control procedures routinely performed with reagent strip testing.
4. name two reasons for measuring urinary pH and discuss their clinical applications.
5. discuss the principle of pH testing by reagent strip.
6. describe three renal causes of proteinuria and two nonrenal reasons for proteinuria.
7. explain the "protein error of indicators" and list any sources of interference that may occur with this method of protein testing.
8. name two confirmatory tests for urine protein performed in the urinalysis laboratory and name any sources of error associated with these procedures.
9. describe the unique solubility characteristics of Bence Jones protein and tell how they can be used to perform a screening test for the presence of this protein.
10. explain why glucose that is normally reabsorbed in the proximal convoluted tubule may appear in the urine.
11. state the renal threshold levels for glucose.
12. describe the principle of the glucose oxidase method of reagent strip testing for glucose and name possible causes of interference with this method.
13. describe the copper reduction method for detection of urinary reducing substances and list possible causes of interference.
14. contrast the advantages and disadvantages of the glucose oxidase and copper reduction methods of glucose testing.
15. name three reasons for the appearance of ketonuria.
16. list the three "ketone bodies" appearing in urine and describe their measurement by the sodium nitroprusside reaction and possible causes of interference.
17. differentiate between hematuria and hemoglobinuria and explain the clinical significance.
18. describe the chemical principle of the reagent strip method for blood testing and list possible causes of interference.

19. discuss the presence of myoglobin and its role in the chemical testing for urinary blood.
20. describe the degradation of hemoglobin to bilirubin, urobilinogen, and finally urobilin.
21. differentiate between conjugated and unconjugated bilirubin, including their relationship to urinary excretion of bilirubin.
22. describe the relationship of urinary bilirubin and urobilinogen to the diagnosis of bile duct obstruction, liver disease, and hemolytic disorders.
23. name the earliest test to detect urinary bilirubin.
24. discuss the principle of oxidation tests and diazotization tests for urinary bilirubin, including possible sources of error.
25. tell the advantage of performing an Ictotest for detection of urine bilirubin.
26. name two technical errors that may produce false-negative bilirubin reactions.
27. give two reasons for increased urine urobilinogen and one reason for an absence of urine urobilinogen.
28. name the chemical contained in Ehrlich's reagent.
29. give the proper method for collecting and preserving specimens to be tested for urine urobilinogen.
30. describe the Watson-Schwartz test used to differentiate among urobilinogen, porphobilinogen, and Ehrlich-reactive compounds.
31. discuss the principle of the nitrite reagent strip test for bacteriuria.
32. List three possible causes of a false-negative result in the reagent strip test for nitrite.
33. compare reagent strip testing for urine specific gravity with urinometer and refractometer testing.
34. give the principle of the reagent strip test for leukocytes.
35. discuss the advantages and disadvantages of the reagent strip test for leukocytes.

REAGENT STRIPS

Routine chemical examination of the urine has changed dramatically since the early days or urine testing, owing to the development of the reagent strip method for chemical analysis. Reagent strips currently provide a simple, rapid means for performing 10 medically significant chemical analyses, including pH, protein, glucose, ketones, blood, bilirubin, urobilinogen, nitrite, specific gravity, and leukocytes. The two major types of dipsticks are manufactured under the tradenames Multistix (Ames Company, Elkhart, IN) and Chemstrip (Bio-Dynamics/BMC, Indianapolis, IN) (Table 4–1). These products are available with single- or multiple-testing areas, and the brand and number of tests used are a matter of laboratory preference. Reagent strips consist of chemical-impregnated absorbent pads attached to a plastic strip. A color-producing chemical reaction takes place when the absorbent pad comes in contact with urine. Color reactions are interpreted by comparing the color produced on the pad with a chart supplied by the manufacturer. Several colors or intensities of a color for each substance being tested appear on the chart. By careful comparison of the colors on the chart and the strip, a semiquantitative value of trace, 1+, 2+, 3+, or 4+ can be reported. An estimate of the milligrams per deciliter present is also available for appropriate testing areas on both products. A summary of chemical testing by reagent strip is provided in Table 4–3, at the conclusion of this chapter.

REAGENT STRIP TECHNIQUE

Testing methodology consists of dipping the strip completely, but briefly, into a well-mixed urine specimen; removing excess urine by touching the edge of the strip to the

TABLE 4–1. Comparison of Reagents and Sensitivity of Multistix and Chemstrip[34, 42]

TEST	MULTISTIX		CHEMSTRIP	
	REAGENTS	SENSITIVITY	REAGENTS	SENSITIVITY
pH	Methyl red Bromthymol blue	pH 5–9	Methyl red Bromthymol blue Phenolphthalein	pH 5–9
Protein	Tetrabromphenol blue	5–20 mg/dl	3′,3″,5′,5″- Tetrachlorophenol- 3,4,5,6- tetrabromosulfophthalein	6 mg/dl
Glucose	Glucose oxidase Peroxidase Potassium iodide	100 mg/dl	Glucose oxidase Peroxidase Tetramethylbenzidine	40 mg/dl
Ketone	Sodium nitroprusside	5–10 mg/dl Acetoacetic acid	Sodium nitroferricyenide Glycine	9 mg/dl Acetoacetic acid 70 mg/dl Acetone
Bilirubin	2, 4-Dichloroaniline diazonium salt	0.2–0.4 mg/dl	2,6-Dichlorobenzene diazonium- tetrafluoroborate	0.5 mg/dl
Blood	Cumene hydroperoxide Tetramethylbenzidine	0.015–0.062 mg/dl Free hemoglobin 5–20 RBCs	Tetramethylbenzidine 2,5-Dimethyl-2,5- dihydroperoxyhexane	5 RBC/μl Hemoglobin from 10 RBC/μl
Urobilinogen	Para-dimethylaminobenzaldehyde	0.1–1.0 Ehrlich units	4-Methoxybenzene- diazonium- tetrafluoroborate	0.4 mg/dl

Test	Reagents			
Nitrite	Para-arsanilic acid 1,2,3,4-Tetrahydrobenzo(h)-quinolin-3-ol	40–80%	3-Hydroxy-1,2,3,4-tetrahydro-7,8-benzoquinoline Sulfanilamide	1% False
Leukocytes	Pyrrole amino acid ester Diazonium salt	5–15 cells/hpf	Indoxycarbonic acid ester Diazonium salt	97.2% Sensitivity
Specific Gravity	Poly(methylvinyl ether maleic anhydride) Bromthymol blue	1.000–1.030		

container as the strip is withdrawn; waiting the specified amount of time for the reaction to occur; and comparing the color of the strip with the color chart. Even though this is a simple procedure, improper technique can result in errors. Allowing the strip to remain in the urine for an extended period of time may cause leaching of reagents from the pads. Likewise, excess urine remaining on the strip after its removal from the specimen can produce a runover between chemicals on adjacent pads, producing distortion of the colors. To ensure against runover, inert absorbent pads have been placed between the affected areas. Holding the strip horizontally while comparing it with the color chart is recommended. The amount of time needed for reactions to take place varies between tests and manufacturers and ranges from an immediate reaction for pH to 120 seconds for leukocytes. For the best semiquantitative results, the manufacturer's stated time should be followed; however, when precise timing cannot be adhered to, it is recommended that reactions be read at 60 seconds but never later than 120 seconds, with the leukocyte reaction read last.[5] A good light source is, of course, essential for accurate interpretations of color reactions.

QUALITY CONTROL AND STORAGE OF REAGENT STRIPS

In addition to the use of correct testing technique, reagent strips must be protected from deterioration caused by moisture, volatile chemicals, heat, and light. Both brands of dipsticks are packaged in opaque containers with desiccant, and when not in use, these bottles should be stored tightly closed in a cool area. Bottles should not be opened in the presence of volatile fumes. All bottles are stamped with an expiration date that represents the functional life expectancy of the chemical pads. This date must be honored even if there is no noticeable deterioration of the reagents. Bottles that have been opened for 6 months should also be discarded regardless of the expiration date. Unexpired strips that have been open for less than 6 months should be visually examined for discoloration and tested for chemical reactivity with controls of known normal and abnormal concentrations. Several commercial controls are available for evaluating reagent strip reactivity, and many methods of preparing and preserving urine specimens of known concentrations have been published.[16] Quality control is as important in urinalysis as it is in other sections of the laboratory and must not be neglected. Personnel from each laboratory shift should test strips from open bottles with both positive and negative controls, compare the values, and record them. A check should also be made whenever a new bottle of reagent strips is opened. Results that do not agree with the published control values must be resolved through the testing of additional reagent strips and controls. Demonstration of chemically acceptable reagent strips does not entirely rule out the possibility of inaccurate results. Interfering substances in the urine, technical carelessness, and color blindness also will produce errors. Both reagent strip manufacturers have published information concerning the limitations of their chemical reactions, and personnel should be aware of these conditions. As mentioned in chapter 3, a primary example of reagent strip interference is the masking of color reactions by the orange pigment present in the urine of persons taking Pyridium compounds. If laboratory personnel do not recognize the presence of this pigment, many erroneous results will be reported. Additional or confirmatory procedures employing different chemical principles must be available for the substances being tested by reagent strip and should be used when questionable results are obtained or, in some instances, to confirm all positive results. The chemical reliability of these procedures must also be checked using positive and negative controls. Specific confirmatory tests and interfering substances are discussed in this chapter under the sections devoted to individual tests.

SUMMARY OF REAGENT STRIP TESTING

Care of Reagent Strips

1. Store with desiccant in an opaque, tightly closed container.
2. Store in a cool place, but do not refrigerate.

3. Do not expose to volatile fumes.
4. Do not use past the expiration date.
5. Use within 6 months after opening.
6. Do not use if chemical pads become discolored.

Technique

1. Mix specimen well.
2. Dip completely, but briefly, into specimen.
3. Remove excess urine when withdrawing strip from specimen.
4. Compare reaction colors with manufacturer's chart under a good light source at the specified time.
5. Perform confirmatory tests when indicated.
6. Be alert for the presence of interfering substances.
7. Understand the principles and significance of the test.
8. Relate chemical findings to each other and to the physical and microscopic urinalysis results.

Quality Control

1. Test open bottles of reagent strips with known positive and negative controls during each laboratory shift.
2. Resolve control results that are out of range by further testing.
3. Test reagents used in confirmatory tests with positive and negative controls.
4. Perform positive and negative controls on new reagents and newly opened bottles of reagent strips.
5. Record all control results and reagent lot numbers.

AUTOMATION IN URINALYSIS

Many studies have been done to determine whether one brand of reagent strip produces fewer errors than the other, and the results have been inconclusive with respect to the quality of the reagent strips. Table 4–1 provides a comparison of the reagents and the sensitivity of the two brands of reagent strips. These same studies have shown that the biggest variable is the conscientiousness of the laboratory personnel in their interpretations of the color reactions.[17] This subjectivity associated with visual discrimination among colors has been alleviated by the development of a semiautomated instrument for the reading of reagent strips. Clini-Tek (Ames Company, Elkhart, IN) measures light reflected from a reagent strip that has been manually dipped in urine and inserted into the machine. Light reflection from the test pads decreases in proportion to the intensity of color produced by the concentration of the test substance.[33] Therefore, the instrument compares the amount of light reflection with that of known concentrations and displays or prints concentration units. An automated instrument for reading reagent strips and performing specific gravity tests utilizes the principle of light reflection for chemical reactions and the falling drop method for specific gravity measurement. The Clinilab (Ames Company, Elkhart, IN) adds urine from vials placed in the machine to the dipsticks, performs the test for specific gravity, and provides printed results. Instrumentation does not improve the chemical methodology of dipsticks, only the reproducibility and color discrimination.[32] Quality control of the reagent strips must also be performed on a regular basis when using automated systems.

Yellow IRIS

The newest addition to automated urinalysis is the Yellow IRIS (International Remote Imaging, Chatsworth, CA 91311), a self-contained, operator-attended work station capable of performing specific gravity tests, routine chemical analysis, and slideless microscopic analysis from an uncentrifuged specimen.

Chemical analysis is performed using an Ames N-Multistix. Urine is poured over the strip as it is poured into the instrument, and the strip is then manually placed into an Ames CliniTek reagent strip reader. Results of the reflectance readings are integrated into the report.

Urine entering the Yellow IRIS is divided into two portions for the specific gravity and microscopic analysis. Specific gravity is determined by analyzing sound-wave frequency. A standard volume of urine is maintained in a U-shaped tube and a sound wave of fixed frequency is transmitted into one end of the tube. The change in frequency recorded as the sound wave exits the other end of the tube is directly related to the specific gravity.

Urine for the microscopic analysis is forced in a moving stream through a sheath of envelope fluid. A process known as planar hydrodynamic positioning forces all particles to flow in a single plane as they pass the optical path of the microscope. Multiple freeze-frame pictures are taken as a particle passes the microscope, and data from these are analyzed by computer as to size and number. Particles are placed into three low-power and five high-power groups based on their size, and the low-power and high-power images are presented to the operator on a color monitor. The operator then makes the final identification by touching an appropriate category on the monitor screen.

Although the Yellow IRIS does require trained personnel to be present when it is running, it does provide the advantages of eliminating the tendency to test urines in batches and allows the operator to perform more analytical than manual tasks.[7] Single-particle analysis will also detect small numbers of constituents that might otherwise be obscured by a predominant element such as the presence of white blood cells in a bloody urine.

pH

Along with the lungs, the kidneys are the major regulators of the acid-base content in the body. They do this through the secretion of hydrogen in the form of ammonium ions, hydrogen phosphate, and weak organic acids, and by the reabsorption of bicarbonate from the filtrate in the convoluted tubules. Although a healthy individual will usually produce a first morning specimen with a slightly acidic pH of 5.0 to 6.0, the pH of normal random samples can range from 4.5 to 8.0. Consequently, there are no normal values assigned to urinary pH, and it must be considered in conjunction with other patient information, such as the acid-base content of the blood, the patient's renal function, the presence of a urinary tract infection, the patient's dietary intake, and the age of the specimen.

CLINICAL SIGNIFICANCE

The importance of urinary pH lies primarily as an aid in determining the existence of systemic acid-base disorders of metabolic or respiratory origin and in the management of urinary conditions that require the urine to be maintained at a specific pH. In respiratory or metabolic acidosis not related to renal function disorders, an acidic urine will be produced; conversely, if respiratory or metabolic alkalosis is present, the urine will be alkaline. Therefore, a urinary pH that does not conform to this pattern may be used to rule out the suspected condition or, as discussed in chapter 2, it may indicate a disorder resulting from the kidneys' inability to secrete or to reabsorb acid or base.

Urinary crystals and renal calculi are formed by the precipitation of inorganic chemicals dissolved in the urine. This precipitation is dependent on urinary pH and can be controlled by maintaining the urine at a pH that is incompatible with the precipitation of the particular chemicals causing the calculi formation. Knowledge of urinary pH is important in the identification of crystals observed during microscopic examination of the urine sediment. This will be discussed in detail in chapter 5.

The maintenance of an acidic urine can be of value in the treatment of urinary tract infections caused by urea-splitting organisms because they do not multiply as readily in an acidic medium. These same organisms are also responsible for the highly alkaline pH found in specimens that have been allowed to sit unpreserved for extended periods of time. Urinary pH is controlled primarily by dietary regulation, although medications may also be used. Persons on high-protein and high-meat diets tend to produce acidic urine; whereas urine from vegetarians is more alkaline owing to the formation of bicarbonate by many fruits and vegetables.[36] An exception to the rule is cranberry juice, which produces an acidic urine and has long been used as a home remedy for minor bladder infections.[22]

SUMMARY OF CLINICAL SIGNIFICANCE OF URINE pH

1. Respiratory or metabolic acidosis
2. Respiratory or metabolic alkalosis
3. Defects in renal tubular secretion and reabsorption of acids and bases
4. Precipitation of crystals and calculi formation
5. Treatment of urinary tract infections
6. Determination of unsatisfactory specimens

Reagent Strip Reactions

Both the Multistix and Chemstrip brands of reagent strips measure urine pH in 1-unit increments between pH 5 and 9. To provide differentiation of pH units throughout this wide range, a double-indicator system of methyl red and bromthymol blue is used by both manufacturers. Methyl red is active in the pH range 4.4 to 6.2, producing a color change from red to yellow; bromthymol blue turns from yellow to blue in the pH range 6.0 to 7.6.[24] Therefore, in the pH range 5 to 9 measured by the dipsticks, one will see colors progressing from orange at pH 5 through yellow and green to a final deep blue at pH 9.

No known substances interfere with urinary pH measurements performed by dipsticks. However, care must be taken to prevent runover between the pH testing area and the adjacent, highly acidic protein testing area, as this may produce a falsely acidic reading in an alkaline urine. Because the pH of freshly excreted urine does not reach a pH of 9 in normal or abnormal conditions, a pH of 9 is associated with an improperly preserved specimen and indicates that a fresh specimen should be obtained to ensure the validity of the analysis.

PROTEIN

Of the routine chemical tests performed on urine, the most indicative of renal disease is the protein determination. The presence of proteinuria is often associated with early renal disease, making the urinary protein test an important part of any physical examination. Normal urine contains very little protein; usually, less than 10 mg/dl or 150 mg per 24 hours is excreted. This protein consists primarily of low-molecular-weight serum proteins that have been selectively filtered by the glomerulus and proteins produced in the genitourinary tract. Due to its low molecular weight, albumin is the major serum protein found in normal urine. However, even though it is present in high concentrations in the plasma, the normal urinary albumin content is low because not all of the albumin presented to the glomerulus is actually filtered, and much of the filtered albumin is reabsorbed by the tubules. Other proteins include small amounts of serum and tubular microglobulins, Tamm-Horsfall protein produced by the tubules, and proteins from prostatic, seminal, and vaginal secretions.

CLINICAL SIGNIFICANCE

Demonstration of proteinuria in a routine analysis does not always signify renal disease; however, its presence does require additional testing to determine whether the protein represents a normal or a pathologic condition. Major pathologic causes of proteinuria include glomerular membrane damage, disorders affecting tubular reabsorption of filtered protein, and increased serum levels of low-molecular-weight proteins. When the glomerular membrane is damaged, selective filtration is impaired, and increased amounts of serum albumin and large globulin molecules pass through the membrane and are excreted in the urine. Conditions that present the glomerular membrane with abnormal substances (e.g., amyloid material, toxic agents, and the immune complexes found in lupus erythematosus and streptococcal glomerulonephritis) are the major causes of proteinuria due to glomerular damage. Increased albumin is also present in disorders that affect tubular reabsorption; however, in contrast to glomerular membrane damage, it is accompanied by other low-molecular-weight proteins of both serum and tubular origin.[21] The amount of protein that appears in the urine following glomerular damage will range from slightly above normal to 40 grams per day; whereas markedly elevated protein levels are seldom seen in tubular disorders.[35]

A primary example of proteinuria due to increased serum protein levels is the excretion of Bence Jones protein by persons with multiple myeloma. In multiple myeloma, a proliferative disorder of the immunoglobulin-producing plasma cells, the serum contains markedly elevated levels of monoclonal immunoglobulin light chains (Bence Jones protein). The low-molecular-weight protein is filtered in quantities exceeding the tubular reabsorption capacity and is excreted in the urine.

Considerable interest is currently being expressed in the measurement of small but consistent amounts of albumin being excreted by diabetic patients. The development of diabetic nephropathy leading to reduced glomerular filtration is a common occurrence in persons with diabetes mellitus. Onset of renal complications can first be predicted by detection of microalbuminuria, and the progression of renal disease can be delayed through better stabilization of blood glucose levels.[43] Immunologic methods are available for measurement of microalbumin and can detect as little as 30 mg/dl.[18]

ORTHOSTATIC (POSTURAL) PROTEINURIA

The discovery of protein, particularly in a random sample, is not always of pathologic significance, inasmuch as several nonrenal or benign causes of proteinuria exist. Benign proteinuria is usually transient and can be produced by conditions such as exposure to cold, strenuous exercise, high fever, dehydration, and in the acute phase of severe illnesses. Proteinuria that occurs during the latter months of pregnancy may indicate a preeclamptic state and should be considered in conjunction with other clinical symptoms to determine whether such a problem exists. Benign proteinuria will disappear when the underlying cause is removed.

A more persistent benign proteinuria occurs frequently in young adults and is termed orthostatic, or postural, proteinuria occurring following periods spent in a vertical posture and disappearing when a horizontal position is assumed. Increased pressure on the renal vein when in the vertical position is believed to account for this condition.[19] Patients suspected of orthostatic proteinuria are requested to collect a specimen immediately upon arising in the morning and a second specimen after remaining in a vertical position for several hours. Both specimens are tested for protein, and if orthostatic proteinuria is present, a negative reading will be seen on the first morning specimen and a positive result will be found on the second specimen.

REAGENT STRIP REACTIONS

Reagent strip testing for protein utilizes the principle of the "protein error of indicators" to produce a visible colorimetric reaction. Contrary to the general belief that indicators produce specific colors in response to particular pH levels, certain indicators change color in the presence or absence of protein even though the pH of the medium remains constant. Depending on the manufacturer, the protein area of the strip contains either tetrabromphenol blue or 3', 3", 5', 5"-tetrachlorophenol-3,4,5,6-tetrabromosulfonphthalein and an acid buffer to maintain the pH at a constant level. At a pH level of 3, both indicators will appear yellow in the absence of protein; however, as the protein concentration increases, the color will progress through various shades of green and finally to blue. Readings are usually reported in terms of negative, trace, 1+, 2+, 3+, and 4+; however, a semiquantitative value in milligrams per deciliter corresponding to each color change is also supplied by the manufacturers. The protein area of reagent strips is one of the most difficult to interpret, particularly in relation to the "trace" reading. For this reason, along with the fact that reagent strips measure primarily albumin and may not detect tubular proteins and Bence Jones protein, most laboratories confirm all positive or questionable protein results with the heat or acid precipitation methods.

A positive test for protein will often be found in conjunction with a positive reaction in the blood portion of the reagent strip and the finding of casts, red blood cells, white blood cells, or bacteria in the microscopic examination. However, it is possible to have a negative protein in the presence of a small number of casts or blood cells.

PRECIPITATION TESTS

The earliest precipitation tests used heat to denature the protein and to produce precipitation; however, other nonprotein substances found in urine are also precipitated by heat. Therefore, acetic acid is added to the heated tube to clear the interfering substances, and sodium chloride is added to ensure protein precipitation in dilute specimens. Currently, most laboratories have replaced the heat and acid test with the less cumbersome cold protein precipitation using sulfosalicylic acid. Various concentrations and amounts of sulfosalicylic acid can be used to precipitate protein, and methods vary greatly among laboratories. By setting up standard curves using known protein concentrations, this method can be adapted to a quantitative procedure, and the amount of precipitation produced can be measured visually against a set of standards or by spectrophotometry or nephelometry. A variety of methods are available for the determination of 24-hour urine protein.[3]

INTERFERING SUBSTANCES

Several substances and conditions produce interference in either the reagent strip or the precipitation method. The major source of error with reagent strips occurs with highly alkaline urine that overrides the buffer system, producing a rise in pH and a color change unrelated to protein concentration. Likewise, a technical error of allowing the reagent pad to remain in contact with the urine for a prolonged period of time may remove the buffer, producing a false-positive reaction. Contamination of the specimen container with quaternary ammonium compounds and detergents may also cause false-positive reactions. High salt concentrations lower the sensitivity of the reagent strip.[14]

Any substance precipitated by acid will, of course, produce false turbidity in the sulfosalicylic acid test. The most frequently encountered substances are radiographic dyes, tolbutamide metabolites, cephalosporins, penicillins, and sulfonamides.[1] The presence of radiographic material can be suspected when a markedly elevated specific gravity is obtained and the precipitate increases on standing but dissolves in acetic acid. The patient's history will provide the necessary information on tolbutamide and antibiotic ingestion. In contrast to the reagent strip test, a highly alkaline urine will produce false-negative readings in precipitation tests as the higher pH interferes with precipitation. All precipitation tests should be performed on centrifuged specimens to remove any extraneous turbidity.

BENCE JONES PROTEIN

When Bence Jones protein is suspected, a screening test that utilizes the unique solubility characteristics of the protein can be performed. Unlike other proteins, which coagulate and remain coagulated when exposed to heat, Bence Jones protein coagulates at temperatures between 40°C and 60°C and dissolves when the temperature reaches 100°C.

Therefore, a specimen that appears turbid between 40°C and 60°C and clear at 100°C can be suspected of containing Bence Jones protein. Interference due to other precipitated proteins can be removed by filtering the specimen at 100°C and observing the specimen for turbidity as it cools to between 40°C and 60°C. Not all persons with multiple myeloma produce detectable Bence Jones protein in the urine, and as mentioned earlier, all suspected cases should have protein and immunoelectrophoresis performed on both serum and urine. Identification of other urinary proteins is also performed in this manner.

SUMMARY OF CLINICAL SIGNIFICANCE OF URINE PROTEIN

1. Glomerular membrane damage
   a. Immune complex disorders
   b. Amyloidosis
   c. Toxic agents
2. Impaired tubular reabsorption
3. Multiple myeloma
4. Orthostatic or postural proteinuria
5. Preeclampsia
6. Diabetic nephropathy

GLUCOSE

Because of its value in the detection and monitoring of diabetes mellitus, the glucose test is the most frequent chemical analysis performed on urine. It is estimated that due to the nonspecific symptoms associated with the onset of diabetes, over half of the cases in the world are undiagnosed.[42] Therefore, urine glucose tests are included in all physical examinations and are often the focus of mass health screening programs. Early diagnosis of diabetes mellitus through blood and urine glucose tests provides a greatly improved prognosis. Using currently available reagent strip and tablet testing methods, patients can monitor themselves at home and can detect regulatory problems prior to the development of serious complications. Patients should be cautioned that diabetic retinopathy can cause misreading, particularly in the blue-green color range.[6]

CLINICAL SIGNIFICANCE

Under normal circumstances, almost all of the glucose filtered by the glomerulus is reabsorbed in the proximal convoluted tubule; therefore, urine contains only minute amounts of glucose. Tubular reabsorption of glucose is by active transport in response to the body's need to maintain an adequate concentration of glucose. Should the blood level of glucose become elevated, as appears in diabetes mellitus, the tubular transport of glucose ceases, and glucose appears in the urine. The blood level at which tubular reabsorption stops is termed the "renal threshold," which for glucose is between 160 and 180 mg per dl. Keep in mind that blood glucose levels will fluctuate, and a normal person may have glycosuria following a meal with a high glucose content. Therefore, the most informative glucose results are obtained from specimens collected under controlled conditions. Fasting prior to the collection of samples for screening tests is recommended. For purposes of diabetes monitoring, specimens are usually tested 2 hours after meals. A first morning specimen does not always represent a fasting specimen because glucose from an evening meal may remain in the bladder overnight, and patients should be advised to empty the bladder and collect the second specimen.[12] Urine for glucose testing is also collected in conjunction with the blood samples drawn during the course of a glucose tolerance test, which is used to confirm the diagnosis of diabetes mellitus.

Glycosuria that is not accompanied by elevated blood glucose levels will be seen

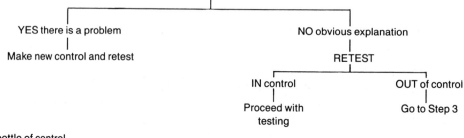

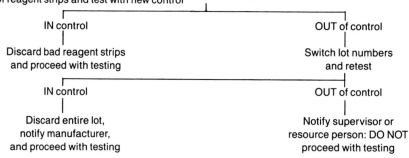

sional epithelial cell attached to a hyaline cast can be expected. However, when tubular damage is present, cells are readily removed from the tubule during cast detachment, and true epithelial cell casts appear in the urine. An entire piece of tubular tissue may be found attached to the cast. Epithelial cell casts are often observed in conjunction with red cell and white cell casts, because both glomerulonephritis and pyelonephritis produce tubular damage. They can be distinguished from white blood cell casts by the presence of a centrally located round nucleus. Identification is aided by staining and phase microscopy **(Color Plates 24 to 26)**.

Granular Casts

The appearance of coarsely and finely granular casts in the urinary sediment is generally considered to represent disintegration of the celluar casts remaining in the tubules as a result of urine stasis **(Color Plate 27)**. Scanning electron microscope studies have confirmed that granular casts seen in conjunction with white blood cell casts contain white cell granules of varying sizes.[24] Bacteria may also be present and can appear as granules under bright-field microscopy. Granular casts unrelated to cellular casts are sometimes seen following periods of stress and strenuous exercise and contain proteins of nonpathologic significance or lysosomes from tubular cells.[17, 18]

Waxy Casts

Previously thought to represent the final disintegration stage of cellular casts, scanning electron microscopy has shown waxy casts to be an advanced stage of the hyaline cast. Examination of the surface ultrastructure shows broken plates of surface protein covering a fibril protein matrix.[17, 23] Waxy casts are refractile with a rigid texture, and this lack of flexibility may cause them to become fragmented as they pass through the tubules **(Color Plates 28 and 29)**.

Fatty Casts

Another disintegration product of cellular casts is the fatty cast, which is produced by the breakdown of epithelial cell casts that contain oval fat bodies. As discussed earlier, renal tubular epithelial cells will absorb lipids entering the tubules through the glomerulus. When these lipid-containing cells become attached to a cast, disintegration produces the fatty cast. Fatty casts are highly refractile and contain yellow-brown fat droplets **(Color Plates 30 and 31)**. A more positive identification can be made by staining with Sudan III or by examining the casts under polarized light.

Broad Casts

As a mold of the distal convoluted tubules, casts may vary in size as disease distorts the tubular structure. Also, when the flow of urine from the tubules to the collecting ducts becomes severely compromised, casts are more likely to form in the collecting ducts. These casts are much larger than other casts and are called broad casts. All types of casts can occur in the broad form, and the finding of many broad waxy casts suggests a serious prognosis **(Color Plates 32 and 33)**. Broad casts are sometimes referred to as renal failure casts. In glomerulonephritis and the nephrotic syndrome, the sediment may contain a wide mixture of the casts and cells just discussed. When this condition is observed, it is termed a telescoped urinary sediment.

BACTERIA

Bacteria are not normally present in the urine. However, unless specimens are collected under sterile conditions, bacterial contamination may occur and is of no clinical significance. Specimens that have remained at room temperature for extended periods of time may also contain noticeable amounts of bacteria that represent nothing more than multiplication of contaminants. Most laboratories report bacteria only when observed in fresh specimens in conjunction with white blood cells **(Color Plate 7)**.

YEAST

Yeast cells, usually *Candida albicans*, may be seen in urine from patients with diabetes mellitus and women with vaginal moniliasis. They are easily confused with red blood cells and should be observed closely for the presence of budding forms **(Color Plates 3 and 27).**

PARASITES

The most frequent parasite encountered in the urine is *Trichomonas vaginalis*, a contaminant from vaginal secretions. The organism is a flagellate and is easily identified by its rapid movement in the microscopic field. However, when not moving, *Trichomonas* may resemble a white blood cell. The ova of a true urinary parasite, *Schistosoma haematobium*, will appear in urine; however, it is seldom seen in the United States. Ova from pinworms and other intestinal parasites are occasionally seen in the urine as a result of fecal contamination.

SPERMATOZOA

Spermatozoa are occasionally found in urine following sexual intercourse or nocturnal emissions and are of no clinical significance **(Color Plate 73).**

MUCUS

Mucus is a protein material produced by glands and epithelial cells in the genitourinary tract. It is not considered clinically significant, and increased amounts usually occur from vaginal contamination. Mucus appears microsopically as threadlike structures with low refractive indexes, requiring observation under subdued light. Care must be taken not to confuse clumps of mucus with hyaline casts. The differentiation can usually be made by observing the irregular appearance of the mucus threads **(Color Plates 16 and 34).**

CRYSTALS

Crystals are frequently found in the urine. Although they are seldom of any clinical significance, identification must be made to ensure that they do not represent an abnormality. Crystals are formed by the precipitation of urine salts subjected to changes in pH, temperature, or concentration, which affect their solubility. The precipitated salts appear in the urine in the form of either true crystals or amorphous material which is also included under the category of urinary crystals.

Normal freshly voided urine may contain crystals formed in the tubules or, less frequently, in the bladder. Increased solute concentration is usually responsible for this invivo precipitation, which is most often encountered in concentrated urine. The majority of crystal formation takes place in specimens that have been allowed to remain at room temperature or that have been refrigerated. Crystals are extremely abundant in refrigerated specimens and often present problems because they obscure other more clinically significant sediment constituents. Some normal crystals will dissolve when the specimen is warmed, but others may require the addition of acid, which will also destroy other formed elements such as red blood cells.

The primary reason for the identification of urinary crystals is to detect the presence of the relatively few abnormal types that may represent such disorders as liver disease, inborn errors of metabolism, or renal damage caused by crystallization of drug metabolites within the tubules.[4]

The most valuable aid in the identification of crystals is knowledge of the urine pH, because this will determine the type of chemicals precipitated. Crystals are routinely categorized not only as normal or abnormal but also by their appearance in acidic or alkaline urine. The most commonly seen crystals have very characteristic shapes or colors; however, variations do occur and can present identification problems, particularly when they resemble abnormal crystals. The identification of crystals in specimens with a neutral pH can also cause difficulty because crystals normally classified as acidic or alkaline types may be found in neutral urine. Normal crystals will be discussed in this chapter with respect to their appearance in acidic or alkaline urine. Abnormal crystals, which are found only in acidic or neutral urine, will be covered in the section after that dealing with normal crystals. The major identifying characteristics of normal crystals are summarized in Table 5–4, and abnormal crystals in Table 5–5.

Normal Crystals

Acid Urine. The most common crystals seen in acidic urine are urates, consisting of uric acid, amorphous urates, and sodium urate. Microscopically, all urate crystals appear yellow to reddish-brown and are the only normal crystals found in acidic urine that appear colored. Uric acid crystals are seen in a variety of shapes, including rhombic plates, rosettes, wedges, and needles. Identification is best made by color rather than by shape. Uric acid crystals show birefringence with polarized light **(Color Plates 35 and 36).** Markedly increased levels of uric acid crystals are seen in leukemia, particularly in those patients receiving chemotherapy, and sometimes in cases of gout. As the name implies, amorphous urates consist of yellow-brown granules, often occurring in clumps that may be confused with granular casts. When present in large amounts, amorphous urates may give the urine—and particularly the sediment—a macroscopic pink color (see chapter 3).

Calcium oxalate crystals are also frequently found in acidic urine, but they can be seen in neutral urine, and even rarely in alkaline urine. In their classic form, they are easily recognized as colorless octahedrals that resemble envelopes; however, dumbbell and oval forms may also occur **(Color Plates 37 and 38).** Calcium oxalate crystals are associated with diets high in oxalic acid and with chemical toxicity and are seen in genetically susceptible persons following large doses of ascorbic acid.[5]

Alkaline Urine. Phosphates represent the majority of the crystals seen in alkaline urine and include triple phosphate, amorphous phosphate, and calcium phosphate. Triple phosphate crystals are probably the most easily identified urine crystals because in their routine form they appear as colorless prisms referred to as "coffin lids" **(Color Plate 39).** They are often seen in large numbers in urine that has been standing at room temperature for several hours. Like amorphous urates, amorphous phosphates are granular in appearance **(Color Plate 40).** When present in large amounts, they produce a macroscopic white turbidity in the urine. Calcium phosphate crystals are not frequently encountered and appear as colorless, thin prisms, plates, or needles. When found in neutral urine, they may be confused with abnormal sulfonamide crystals; however, calcium phosphate crystals are soluble in dilute acetic acid, and sulfonamides are not.

Other normal crystals associated with alkaline urine are ammonium biurate and calcium carbonate. Like the urate crystals, ammonium biurate crystals have a yellow-brown color. They are frequently described as "thorny apples" due to their appearance as spicule-covered spheres. Calcium carbonate crystals are small and colorless, with dumbbell or spherical shapes. They may occur in clumps that resemble amorphous phosphates, but they can be distinguished by the formation of gas after the addition of acetic acid.

Abnormal Crystals

The abnormal crystals of primary concern include cystine, cholesterol, leucine, tyrosine, sulfonamides, radiographic dyes, and ampicillin. Hemosiderin, appearing as yellow-brown granules, may also be seen in anemias caused by red blood cell destruction. The granules are sometimes located in casts and epithelial cells but are also free floating. Staining the sediment with Prussian blue will confirm the presence of hemosiderin. Use of the cytocentrifuge to obtain well-fixed slides with intact renal tubular epithelial cells aids in the identification.[32]

Most abnormal crystals have characteristic shapes, all are found in acid or neutral

TABLE 5–4. Major Characteristics of Normal Urinary Crystals[4]

CRYSTAL	pH	COLOR	SOLUBILITY	APPEARANCE
Uric acid	Acid	Yellow-brown	Alkali soluble	
Amorphous urates	Acid	Brick dust or yellow brown	Alkali and heat	
Calcium oxalate	Acid/neutral (alkaline)	Colorless (envelopes)	Dilute HCl	
Amorphous phosphates	Alkaline Neutral	White-colorless	Dilute acetic acid	
Calcium phosphate	Alkaline Neutral	Colorless	Dilute acetic acid	
Triple phosphate	Alkaline	Colorless (coffin lids)	Dilute acetic acid	
Ammonium biurate	Alkaline	Yellow-brown (thorny apples)	Acetic acid with heat	
Calcium carbonate	Alkaline	Colorless (dumbbells)	Gas from acetic acid	

TABLE 5–5. Major Characteristics of Abnormal Urinary Crystals[4]

CRYSTAL	pH	COLOR	SOLUBILITY	APPEARANCE
Cystine	Acid	Colorless	Ammonia, dilute HCl	
Cholesterol	Acid	Colorless (notched plates)	Chloroform	
Leucine	Acid/neutral	Yellow	Hot alkali or alcohol	
Tyrosine	Acid/neutral	Colorless-yellow	Alkali or heat	
Bilirubin	Acid	Yellow	Acetic acid, HCl, NaOH, ether, chloroform	
Sulfonamides	Acid/neutral	Green	Acetone	
Radiographic dye	Acid	Colorless	10% NaOH	
Ampicillin	Acid/neutral	Colorless	Refrigeration forms bundles	

urine, and chemical tests are available for positive identification. Cystine crystals that appear as colorless hexagonal plates are found in persons who inherit a metabolic defect that prevents the reabsorption of cystine by the proximal convoluted tubule (**Color Plate 41**). Persons with cystinuria have a tendency to form renal calculi. Cholesterol crystals are rarely seen unless specimens have been refrigerated, because the lipids remain in droplet form. However, when observed, they have a most characteristic appearance, resembling a rectangular plate with a notch in one or more corners (**Color Plates 42 and 43**).

Leucine crystals, which appear as yellow-brown spheres that contain concentric circles with radial striations, and tyrosine crystals, which resemble sheaths of fine needles, are seen rarely in cases of severe liver disease (**Color Plate 44**). Also seen in liver disease are bilirubin crystals, appearing as clumped needles or granules with characteristic yellow color (**Color Plate 45**).

Until the development of more soluble sulfonamides, the appearance of these crystals in urine was common in patients who were not adequately hydrated. This condition could result in tubular damage if crystals formed in the nephron. Likewise, patients exhibiting radiographic dye and ampicillin crystals may develop problems if sufficient fluid is not taken. Radiographic dye crystals may resemble uric acid but can be suspected in specimens that have an abnormally high specific gravity. Ampicillin crystals appear as needles that form bundles after refrigeration (**Color Plate 46**).

As discussed earlier, the use of polarized light also can aid in crystal identification. The problems associated with the identification of abnormal crystals can often be solved by a check on the medications and treatments the patient is receiving. When this is not done, considerable time and energy can be wasted trying to identify the crystals solely by appearance.

RENAL CALCULI

Numerous correlation studies between the presence of crystalluria and the formation of renal calculi have been conducted with varying results. The finding of clumps of crystals in freshly voided, warm urine suggests that conditions may be right for calculus formation, and increased crystalluria has been noted during the summer months in persons who form kidney stones.[19] However, due to variation in conditions that affect urine within the body and in the specimen container and the fact that a true understanding of the mechanisms of calculi formation is not available, little importance is placed on the role of crystals in the diagnosis of renal calculi.[3]

Analysis of passed renal calculi is an important aid in patient management. Approximately 75 percent of the calculi contain calcium oxalate, and future formations may be prevented by dietary changes. Analysis of calculi can be performed chemically, but examination by x-ray crystallography provides a more comprehensive analysis.[26]

ARTIFACTS

Contaminants of all types can be found in urine, particularly in those specimens collected under improper conditions or in dirty containers. Most confusing to students are oil droplets and starch granules (talcum powder), because they resemble red blood cells (**Color Plates 4 and 47**). However, they are much more refractile, and if polarized light is used, starch granules will exhibit Maltese-cross formation. Addition of dilute acetic acid will dissolve red blood cells, leaving yeast and oil droplets intact. Hair and other fibers may initially be mistaken for casts, but close examination should rule this out (**Color Plate 48**).

QUALITY ASSURANCE IN URINALYSIS

During the discussion of the routine urinalysis in this and the preceding two chapters, the methods of ensuring accurate test results were covered on an individual basis for each of the tests. Because quality control in the urinalysis laboratory—or any other laboratory department—is an integration of many factors, this section will provide an overall view of the procedures essential for providing quality urinalysis.

Total quality control has been categorized in many ways. Table 5–6 shows a comparison between the original industrial quality-control measurements and laboratory quality control. Plaut and Silberman[30] outline the system in the following manner:

1. Sample collection and identification
2. Methodology
    Instrumentation
    Reagents
    Calibration
3. Instrument maintenance
    Manufacturer's recommendations
    Laboratory preventive maintenance
4. Quality control
    Material
    Data handling

To each of these outlines should also be added training and continuing education of the personnel performing the tests.

Documentation of quality-control procedures is essential for laboratory accreditation by either the Joint Commission of Accreditation of Hospitals (JCAH) or the College of American Pathologists (CAP) and for Medicare approval. Guidelines published by CAP provide very complete instructions for documentation and are used as a reference for the ensuing discussion of the specific areas of urinalysis quality control.[8]

SUPERVISION OF QUALITY CONTROL

The urinalysis section supervisor or a designated person should monitor the quality-control results, and the program is reviewed monthly by the pathologist or laboratory quality-control supervisor. Records should be available for all shifts, covering controls

TABLE 5–6. Comparison between Original Industrial Quality Control Measurements and Laboratory Quality Control*

	IN INDUSTRY	MEDICAL LABORATORY
Phase I.	New design control	Selection of the proper tests and the proper method for a particular patient problem
Phase II.	Incoming material control	Standards, control sera, and evaluation of reagent kits and instruments, and so forth
Phase III.	Process control	Internal quality control and external quality control (proficiency testing)
Phase IV.	Product output control	Format of presentation of results to physicians to solve a patient problem
Phase V.	Product reliability	Reliability of the interpretation of the result by the physician
Phase VI.	Special process studies	An inspection and accreditation program

*From Eilers,[10] p 1364, with permission.

TABLE 5–7. Reporting Results/Reviewing Results/Correction of Errors*

1. Early AM urinalysis results on ICU and CCU should be completed and telephoned to the respective units by 10 AM.

2. STAT urinalysis should be completed and called within 30 minutes of collection.

3. On preoperative urinalysis, notify the patient's physician or charge nurse of abnormal results as soon as possible so that another specimen can be obtained and tested prior to surgery. This is particularly important for outpatients scheduled for surgery.

4. At least once each shift, the hematology supervisor or charge technician will review all urinalysis reports for clarity.

5. If an error in reporting has been made or results are questioned, the test will be repeated on the same sample, if available. If the specimen is no longer available and repeat testing is indicated, ask for another specimen and retest.

6. Correction of errors: If an incorrect result has been posted to the patient's chart, *do not remove the report*. Mark an X through the erroneous result and post the corrected result, so labeled, on a new reporting form in the patient's chart near the invalid result. This should be handled by the supervisor or charge technician.

*From Patricia Stirk, MT (ASCP), Fair Oaks Hospital Department of Pathology,[11] with permission.

and instrument checks. Written procedures for detection and correction of errors, out-of-control results, and review of test results are necessary (see Table 5–7).

PROCEDURE MANUAL

A procedure manual containing all of the procedures performed in the urinalysis section must be available for reference in the working area. The following information is included for each procedure: specimen handling, test principles, preparation of reagents, controls and standards, methodology, calculations, tolerance limits for controls, normal values, special requirements, and references. Package inserts may be included but should not replace a carefully written procedure that includes specific laboratory information.

Evaluation of new procedures and adoption of new methodologies is an ongoing process in the clinical laboratory. All changes in the procedure manual are initialed by the section supervisor, and the manual must be reviewed annually by the laboratory director (see Table 5–8).

SPECIMEN HANDLING

As discussed in chapter 1, all specimens should be examined fresh. If this is not possible, written instructions for the preservation of specimens for both routine and special procedures must be available. A policy such as the one shown in Table 5–9 should be available for mislabeled specimens.

REAGENTS

All reagents and reagent strips must be properly labeled with the date of preparation or opening, purchase date, and expiration date. Reagent strips should be checked against a known control solution on each shift and whenever a new bottle is opened. Reagents are checked daily or when tests requiring their use are requested. Results of all reagent checks are recorded.

Many commercial control materials are available for monitoring reagent and reagent strip reactivity; however, most do not include sediment constituents for monitoring the microscopic analysis. Controls for nitrite and leukocyte esterase can be prepared by making aliquots of positive patient specimens and storing them in the refrigerator for 1 week.

In-house controls, as described in Table 5–10, provide an inexpensive way to monitor performance. Preparation of controls containing sediment constituents can be done using a method described by Hoeltge and Ersts.[20] Elements to be preserved are washed

TABLE 5–8. Urine Normal Ranges*

CONSTITUENT	FINDINGS
Specific gravity	1.001–1.035
Volume, average 24 hour	1,200–1,500 ml
Volume, outer range of normal	600–2,000 ml
pH range	4.7–8.0 average 6
Ketones	negative
Glucose	negative
Clinitest	negative
Protein	negative to trace
Bilirubin	negative
Urobilinogen	less than 1 mg/dl
WBC esterase	negative
Nitrite	negative
Occult blood	negative
MICROSCOPIC FINDINGS	
WBC	0–3
RBC	0–3
Epithelial cells	only squamous
Crystals	few calcium oxalate, few amorphous urates or phosphates
Mucus	less than 1 +
Casts	0–1 hyaline casts
Bacteria	few HPF or less than 1 +
Yeast	negative
Trichomanads	negative

References:
1. BioDynamics Chemistrip 9: 1983, BioDynamics: Diagnostic Test Values, pages 10–37.
2. Urinalysis and Body Fluids; Susan King Strasinger, 1985 F.A. Davis Co., pages 3, 50, 98, 99, 95–98, 93, 94.
3. Todd & Sanford, p. 577, Medical Microscopy and Examination of Other Body Fluids, 1979, W.B. Saunders, Co.

GENESIS: 11-29-86 - PS

*From Fair Oaks Hospital,[11] with permission.

TABLE 5–9. Policy for Handling Mislabeled Specimens*

Do NOT assume any information about the specimen or patient.
Do NOT relabel an incorrectly labeled specimen.
Do NOT discard the specimen until investigation is complete.
Leave specimen EXACTLY as you receive it; put in the refrigerator for preservation until errors can be resolved.
Notify floor, nursing station, Dr's office, etc., of problem and why it must be corrected for analysis to continue.
Identify problem on specimen requisition with date, time, and your initials.
Make person responsible for specimen collection participate in solution of problem(s). Any action taken should be documented on the requisition slip.
Report all mislabeled specimens to the quality assurance board.

*From Schweitzer, Schumann, and Schumann,[41] p 568, with permission.

TABLE 5–10. The Mount Vernon Hospital Chemistry Lab—Urinalysis Quality Control*

I. Perform the following DAILY.
  1. Clean the work area with disinfectant.
  2. Refractometer: read specific gravity of water—1.000
                    read specific gravity of 5% NaCl—should read 1.022 ± .001
  3. Harleco URINTROL (may be stored at room temperature after opening—mix thoroughly by gently inverting 10–15 times):
    a. Specific gravity—refractometer
    b. Chemstrip 9
    c. Sulfosalicylic acid
    d. Clinitest
  4. All results are recorded on the quality control forms, and initialed.
  5. When a test is out of control
    a. DO NOT REPORT OUT RESULTS
    b. Check reagents for contamination, outdating, and/or correct lot numbers
    c. Repeat using new Urintrol and fresh reagents
    d. Notify supervisor
  6. Daily in-house control:

    Each day, the morning shift will choose one urine specimen of sufficient quantity for the in-house control for that day. Each of the following two shifts will also do a complete urinalysis (including microscopic) on this same specimen. Store in the refrigerator when not in use. Allow specimen to come to room temperature before use.

    Record results on the In-House Control Forms in the notebook for the appropriate shift.

II. Perform the following AS REQUIRED. Do only when (a) a patient test is required and (b) it has not been done that day.
  1. Harleco Urintrol
    a. Acetest
    b. Ictotest
    c. Chemstrip GK
  2. Record all results on the Quality Control Form, and initial.

TABLE 5–10. *continued*

III. Perform the following WEEKLY.

1. Clean and check sulfosalicylic acid dispenser:

   Volumetrically pipette 1.0 ml sulfosalicylic acid into a 10-ml volumetric flask. Make sure the Oxford Pipettor is primed, and dispense three 3.0-ml aliquots into the volumetric flask. This should equal 10.0 ml. If not, adjust the pipettor accordingly and recheck.

   Log under Miscellaneous Quality Control, and initial.

2. Read the pH on the Chemstrip 9 after dipping the strip in the pH 7 buffer (pH meter buffer).

   This should read 6.5–7.5. Record under Miscellaneous on Quality Control Forms, and initial.

3. Check pH of distilled water using pH meter. Record and initial sheet on the wall in the dishwashing room and by the chemistry spigot. Also check the resistance of both water supplies and record.

4. Clean the centrifuge with disinfectant.

IV. Perform the following MONTHLY.

1. Make certain that Microbiology has cultured both water supplies and that the bacterial count is below 100 organisms/ml for each.

---

*From Clare Bowman, MT (ASCP), Mount Vernon Hospital Department of Pathology,[28] with permission.

in cold 0.85 percent saline and fixed overnight in a 10 percent formalin-saline solution (0.85 g sodium chloride plus 10 ml aqueous formalin, q.s. to 100 ml with distilled water). Aliquots added to chemical controls can then be frozen.

External quality-control programs such as that offered by the CAP provide an additional means for monitoring laboratory quality. Laboratories subscribing to this program receive lyophilized specimens for routine urinalysis and transparencies for sediment constituent identification every 3 months. The results are returned to the CAP, where they are statistically analyzed with those from all participating laboratories, and a report is returned to the laboratory director. Corrective action must be taken for unacceptable results.

Corrective action, including the use of new reagents or reagent strips and controls and the verification of lot numbers and expiration dates, must be taken when control values are outside the tolerance limits. All corrective actions taken are documented. A protocol for corrective action is shown in Figure 5–1.

INSTRUMENTATION AND EQUIPMENT

The most frequently encountered instruments in the urinalysis laboratory are those used to measure urine solute. They include urinometers, refractometers, and osmometers. Both urinometers and refractometers are calibrated daily against distilled water (1.000) and a known control, such as 5 percent saline (1.022 ± 0.001) or 9 percent sucrose (1.034 ± 0.001). Both high and low commercial controls are available for the osmometer. All control values are recorded.

Automated urinalysis systems and reagent strip readers are calibrated using negative and positive controls.

Equipment found in the urinalysis laboratory includes primarily refrigerators, centrifuges, microscopes, and water baths. Temperatures of refrigerators and water baths

A. Record all actions taken and the resolution of any problems

B. Use the flow diagram below:

    1. Run control

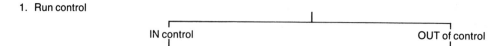

    2. Inspect control for: Outdate (age), proper storage, correct lot number, signs of contamination.

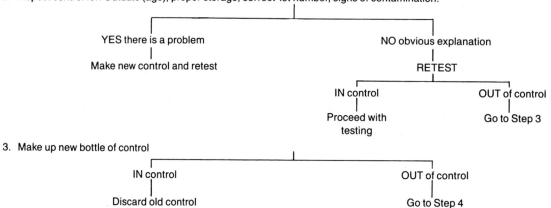

    3. Make up new bottle of control

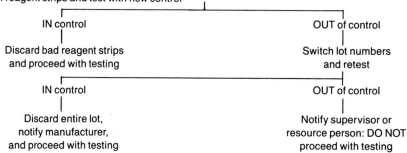

    4. Open new can of reagent strips and test with new control

IN control	OUT of control
Discard bad reagent strips and proceed with testing	Switch lot numbers and retest

IN control	OUT of control
Discard entire lot, notify manufacturer, and proceed with testing	Notify supervisor or resource person: DO NOT proceed with testing

FIGURE 5–1. "Out of control" procedures. (From J Med Technol 3:11, 1986; J Med Technol 48(2):571, 1986, with permission.)

should be taken daily and recorded. Calibration of centrifuges is customarily performed every 3 months, and the appropriate RCF for each setting is recorded. A routine maintenance schedule for each piece of equipment should be prepared, and records should be kept of all routine and nonroutine maintenance performed. Deionized water used for reagent preparation is quality controlled by checking pH, purity meter resistance, and bacterial count.

    Table 5–10 provides a daily, weekly, and monthly description of routine quality-control procedures in the urinalysis laboratory.

REPORTING OF RESULTS

Forms for reporting results should provide adequate space for writing and should present the information in a logical sequence. Standardized reporting methods will minimize physician confusion in interpreting results (see Table 5–11). Review of the report slips by the section supervisor on a periodic basis throughout the shift will aid in detecting

**TABLE 5–11. The Mount Vernon Hospital Routine Urinalysis Standardization
of Report**

1. Color

   Yellow, dark yellow, bright yellow, or other colors (owing to medication)

2. Appearance

   Clear, slightly hazy, hazy, cloudy, turbid

3. Reaction to Chemstrip 9 and other chemical tests.

   a. Protein: negative, trace, 1+, 2+, 3+, 4+ (back-up test: Sulfa Sal)
   b. Glucose: negative, trace, 1+, 2+, 3+, 4+ (back-up test: Clinitest)*
   c. Ketones: negative, trace, 1+, 2+, 3+ (back-up test: Acetest)
   d. Urobilinogen: normal, 1, 4, 8, 12 mg/dl
   e. Bilirubin: negative, trace, 1+, 2+, 3+ (back-up test: Ictotest)
   f. Blood: negative, trace, 1+, 2+ 3+
   g. Leukocytes: trace, 1+, 2+
   h. Nitrites: negative, positive

   A back-up test, when available, is performed on all questionable Chemstrip 9 tests. The result of the dipstick test, if confirmed, is the one reported out, and the back-up test(s) performed is recorded on the log-in sheet.

4. Microscopic examination

   a. Leukocytes: record average number per high-power field
   b. Erythrocytes: record average number per high-power field
   c. Epithelial cells

      Rare: 1 in every five high-powered fields
      Occ.: 1 in every high-powered field
      Few: 2–5 in every high-powered field
      Mod: 5–10 in every high-powered field
      Many: 10 or more in every high-powered field

   d. Mucous threads: light, moderate, heavy
   e. Crystals: report the same as for epithelial cells
   f. Amorphous material: light, moderate, heavy
   g. Bacteria: report as negative, light, moderate, heavy
   h. Casts: identify type per *low*-powered field
      Report number present per low-power field

Centrifuge 10 ml urine for 5 minutes at 400 G (1500 RPM) (set at 3 on Sorvall)

---

   *Also check urine of all patients under 2 years old for reducing substances using Clinitest tablets.

errors and will provide for their timely correction. Written procedures should be available for the reporting of critical values (see Table 5–12). In laboratories analyzing pediatric specimens this should include the presence of ketosis or sugars in newborns.

Personnel and Facilities

Quality control is only as good as the personnel performing and monitoring it. Personnel must understand the importance of quality assurance, and the program should be administered in a manner such that personnel view it as a learning experience rather than as a threat.[41] Up-to-date reference materials and atlases should be readily available in the section, and documentation of continuing education maintained.

TABLE 5–12. Urinalysis Panic Values—Notification of Doctor or Charge Nurse*

Notify the doctor or charge nurse if any of the following occur:

Positive glucose and/or Clinitest 2% or higher
Positive bilirubin/Ictotest
Many granular casts, WBC or RBC casts, or waxy casts
Positive protein/SSA greater than 3+ to 4+ range
Unusual crystals such as cystine

*From Patricia Stirk, MT (ASCP), Fair Oaks Hospital Department of Pathology,[11] with permission.

An adequate, uncluttered, safe working area is also essential for both quality work and personnel morale. Universal precautions for handling body fluids should be followed at all times.

REFERENCES

1. Addis, T: The number of formed elements in the urinary sediment of normal individuals. J Clin Invest 2(5):409–415, 1926.
2. Berham, L and O'Kell, RT: Urinalysis: Minimizing microscopy. Clin Chem 28(7):1722, 1982.
3. Boyce, WH: Calculous disease: Guest editorial. J Urol 127(5):859, 1982.
4. Bradley, M and Schumann, GB: Examination of the urine. In Henry, JB (ed): Clinical Diagnosis and Management by Laboratory Methods. WB Saunders, Philadelphia, 1984.
5. Bradley, M: Urine crystals: Identification and significance. Lab Med 13(6):348–353, 1982.
6. Brody, L, Webster, MC, and Kark, RM: Identification of elements in the urinary sediment with phase-contrast microscopy. JAMA 206(8):1777–1781, 1968.
7. Cannon, DC: The identification and pathogenesis of urine casts. Lab Med 10(1):8–11, 1979.
8. College of American Pathologists: Commission of Inspection and Accreditation Inspection Checklist. Section 111A: Urinalysis. College of American Pathologists, Skokie, IL, 1987.
9. Dudas, H: Quality in urinalysis. Lab Med 12(12):765–767, 1981.
10. Eilers, RJ: Total quality control for the medical laboratory. South Med J 62(11):1362–1365, 1969.
11. Fair Oaks Hospital: Department of Pathology Quality Control Procedure. Fairfax, VA, 1988.
12. Fassett, RG, et al: Urinary red cell morphology during exercise. Am J Clin Pathol 285(6353):1455–1457, 1982.
13. Ferris, JA: Comparison and standardization of the urine microscopic examination. Lab Med 14(10):659–662, 1983.
14. Fletcher, AP, Neuberger, A, and Ratcliffe, WA: Tamm-Horsfall urinary glycoprotein: The chemical composition. Biochem J 120:417–424, 1970.
15. Haber, MH: Urinary Sediment: A Textbook Atlas. American Society of Clinical Pathologists, Chicago, 1981.
16. Haber, MH: Interference contrast microscopy for identification of urinary sediments. Am J Clin Pathol 57:316–319, 1972.
17. Haber, MH and Lindner, LE: The surface ultrastructure of urinary casts. Am J Clin Pathol 68(5):547–552, 1977.

18. Haber, MH, Lindner, LE, and Ciofalo, LN: Urinary casts after stress. Lab Med 10(6):351–355, 1979.
19. Hallson, PC and Rose, GA: Seasonal variations in urinary crystals. Br J Urol 49(4):277–284, 1977.
20. Hoeltge, GA and Ersts, BS: A quality control system for the general urinalysis laboratory. Am J Clin Pathol 73(3):403–408, 1980.
21. Kark, RM: A Primer of Urinalysis. Harper & Row, New York, 1963.
22. ICL Scientific: KOVA System for Standardized Urinalysis. Fountain Valley, CA, 1981.
23. Lindner, LE and Haber, MH: Hyaline casts in the urine: Mechanism of formation and morphological transformations. Am J Clin Pathol 80(3):347–352, 1983.
24. Lindner, LE, Vacca, D, and Haber, MH: Identification and composition of types of granular urinary casts. Am J Clin Pathol 80(3):353–358, 1983.
25. Lindner, LE, Jones, RN, and Haber, MH: A specific cast in acute pyelonephritis. Am J Clin Pathol 73(6):809–811, 1980.
26. Mandel, N: Urinary tract calculi. Lab Med 17(8):449–458, 1986.
27. McGuchen, M, Cohen, L, and MacGregor, RR: Significance of pyuria in urinary sediment. J Urol 120:452–456, 1978.
28. Mount Vernon Hospital: Department of Pathology Quality Control Procedure. Alexandria, VA, 1988.
29. Mynahan, C: Evaluation of macroscopic urinalysis as a screening procedure. Lab Med 15(3):176–179, 1984.
30. Plaut, D and Silberman, J: Quality control in the automated laboratory. Am J Med Technol 49(4):213–218, 1983.
31. Product Profile: Sedi-Stain. Clay Adams, Division of Becton, Dickinson & Company, Parsippany, NJ, 1974.
32. Ritz, L and Krushall, M: An improved urine hemosiderin procedure using cytocentrifugation. Lab Med 17(5):102, 1986.
33. Schreiner, GE and Welt, LG: Diseases of the Kidney. Little, Brown & Co, Boston, 1963.
34. Schumann, GB and Greenberg, NF: Usefulness of macroscopic urinalysis as a screening procedure. Am J Clin Pathol 71(6):452–454, 1979.
35. Schumann, GB, Henry, JB, and Harris, S: An improved technique for examining urinary casts and a review of their significance. Am J Clin Pathol 69:18–23, 1978.
36. Schumann, GB, Schumann, JL, and Schweitzer, SC: The urine sediment examination: a coordinated approach. Lab Man 21:45–48, 1983.
37. Schumann, GB and Tebbs, RD: Comparison of slides used for standardized routine microscopic urinalysis. J Med Technol 3(1):54–58, 1986.
38. Smalley, DL and Bryan, JA: Comparative evaluation of biochemical and microscopic urinalysis. Am J Med Technol 49(4):237–239, 1983.
39. Stapleton, FB: Morphology of urinary red blood cells: A simple guide in localizing the site of hematuria. Pediatr Clin N Am 34(3):561–569, 1987.
40. Sternheimer, R and Malbin, R: Clinical recognition of pyelonephritis with a new stain for urinary sediments. Am J Med 11:312–313, 1951.
41. Schweitzer, SC, Schumann, JL, and Schumann, GB: Quality assurance guidelines for the urinalysis laboratory. J Med Technol 3(11):567–572, 1986.
42. Szwed, JJ and Schaust, C: The importance of microscopic examination of the urinary sediment. Am J Med Technol 48(2):141–143, 1982.
43. Thal, SM et al: Comparison of dysmorphic erythrocytes with other urinary sediment parameters of renal bleeding. Am J Clin Pathol 86(6):784–787, 1986.
44. Yu, HD: Evaluation of microscopic examination of bacteriuria. Chinese Journal of Microbiology 11(1):16–20, 1978.

STUDY QUESTIONS (Choose one best answer)

1. Correct performance of a urinary sediment examination should include
   1. centrifugation of 10 ml of urine for 5 minutes
   2. addition of preservative prior to centrifugation
   3. resuspending the sediment in 0.5 ml of urine
   4. examining under low and high power
   5. reporting all constituents as number per high-power field
   a. 1, 2, and 3
   b. 2, 4, and 5
   c. 1, 3, and 4
   d. 1, 3, and 5

2. The predecessor of the standardized urine microscopic examination was the
   a. Sternheimer count
   b. Addis count
   c. Kova system
   d. T-system

3. For better detection of hyaline casts, bright-field microscopy can be replaced by
   a. phase-contrast microscopy
   b. polarized light
   c. compensated polarized light
   d. dark-field microscopy

4. Identification of oval fat bodies can be made using
   a. bright-field microscopy
   b. phase contrast
   c. polarized light
   d. interference-contrast microscopy

5. In order to observe elements with a low refractive index when using bright-field microscopy, the
   a. condenser is raised to increase light
   b. condenser is lowered to increase light
   c. condenser is raised to reduce light
   d. condenser is lowered to reduce light

6. Relative centrifugal force (RCF) is determined by which two factors?
   a. radius of rotor head and RPM
   b. radius of rotor head and time of centrifugation
   c. diameter of rotor head and RPM
   d. RPM and time of centrifugation

7. Which of the following elements would most likely be found in an acidic concentrated urine that contains protein?
   a. ghost red blood cells
   b. casts
   c. bacteria
   d. triple phosphate crystals

8. Urinary sediment from a patient suspected of having renal calculi should contain
   a. white blood cells
   b. casts
   c. red blood cells
   d. triple phosphate crystals

9. Differentiation among red blood cells, yeast, and oil droplets may be accomplished by all of the following except

   a. observation of budding in yeast cells
   b. increased refractibility of oil droplets
   c. lysis of yeast cells by acetic acid
   d. lysis of red blood cells by acetic acid

10. A positive chemical test for blood with no red blood cells found in the sediment

   a. should have both tests repeated if the specimen is clear and red
   b. indicates the presence of hemoglobin or myoglobin
   c. indicates possible acute glomerulonephritis
   d. is not possible

11. Ghost red blood cells are seen in

   a. dilute acidic urine
   b. dilute alkaline urine
   c. concentrated acidic urine
   d. concentrated alkaline urine

12. An increase in urinary white blood cells is called

   a. pyelonephritis
   b. cystitis
   c. urethritis
   d. pyuria

13. Leukocytes that stain pale blue with Sternheimer-Malbin stain and exhibit brownian movement are

   a. indicative of pyelonephritis
   b. basophils
   c. mononuclear leukocytes
   d. glitter cells

14. Oval fat bodies are

   a. squamous epithelial cells that contain lipids
   b. renal tubular epithelial cells that contain lipids
   c. free-floating fat droplets
   d. white blood cells with phagocytized lipids

15. Damage to the glomerular membrane can be suspected when the sediment contains

   a. hyaline casts
   b. red blood cell casts
   c. waxy casts
   d. epithelial cell casts

16. The matrix of casts consists of

   a. filtered protein
   b. fatty deposits
   c. Tamm-Horsfall protein
   d. cellular debris

17. Broad casts are

   a. formed by the disintegration of waxy and fatty casts
   b. formed in the distal convoluted tubules instead of the proximal convoluted tubules
   c. formed at the juncture of the ascending loop of Henle
   d. formed in the collecting ducts

18. A urine specimen refrigerated overnight is cloudy and has a pH of 8. The turbidity is probably due to

    a. amorphous phosphates
    b. amorphous urates
    c. triple phosphate crystals
    d. calcium oxalate crystals

19. To confirm the above identification, you could

    a. warm the specimen
    b. add sodium hydroxide
    c. add dilute hydrochloric acid
    d. add dilute acetic acid

20. Normal crystals found in acidic urine include

    a. calcium oxalate, uric acid, amorphous urates
    b. calcium oxalate, uric acid, sulfonamides
    c. uric acid, amorphous urates, calcium carbonate
    d. uric acid, calcium carbonate, ammonium biurate

21. Name a crystal that matches the following descriptions:

    a. "coffin-lid"   _____
    b. "thorny apple"   _____
    c. "envelope"   _____
    d. "dumbbell"   _____

22. Match the following crystals:

    ____ cholesterol   a. spherical, with concentric circles with
    ____ leucine   radial striations
    ____ cystine   b. sheaths of fine needles
    ____ tyrosine   c. Maltese cross
                                  d. notched corners
                                  e. hexagonal plates

23. As supervisor of the urinalysis laboratory, you have just adopted a new procedure. You should

    a. put the package insert in the procedure manual
    b. put a complete, referenced procedure in the manual
    c. notify the microbiology department
    d. put a cost analysis study in the procedure manual

24. Deionized water used for the preparation of reagents should be checked for

    a. calcium content
    b. bacterial content
    c. filter contamination
    d. pH, purity, and bacteria

25. While working on the evening shift, you receive a specimen and a requisition slip that do not match. You should

    a. notify the nursing station to correct the error
    b. notify the nursing station and proceed with testing
    c. discard the specimen immediately
    d. refrigerate the specimen for the day shift

26. The following results were obtained on a urine specimen from a 30-year-old woman:

    Color: brown   Ketone: negative
    Appearance: cloudy   Bilirubin: negative
    Sp. Gr.: 1.027   Urobilinogen: 0.1 EU
    pH: 5.5   Blood: moderate
    Protein: 2 +   Nitrite: positive
    Glucose: negative

    Indicate if these results suggest that any of the following may be seen in the sediment and support your answer:

    a. RBCs
    b. WBCs
    c. casts
    d. bacteria

27. A 22-year-old female college student comes to the university health center complaining of a burning sensation while voiding. The urinalysis shows:

    Color: straw   Ketone: negative
    Appearance: hazy   Bilirubin: negative
    Sp. Gr.: 1.008   Urobilinogen: 0.1 EU
    pH: 8.0   Blood: trace
    Protein: trace   Nitrite: positive
    Glucose: negative

    Indicate if these results suggest that any of the following may be seen in the sediment and support your answer:

    a. RBCs
    b. WBCs
    c. crystals
    d. bacteria

28. A medical technology student performs a urinalysis on himself after completing a marathon run. The results are the following:

    Color: dark   Urobilinogen: 1.0 EU
    Appearance: clear   Blood: small
    Sp. Gr.: 1.030   Nitrite: negative
    pH: 5.5   Leukocyte esterase: negative
    Protein: 2 +   0–4 hyaline casts/lpf
    Glucose: negative   0–5 WBC/hpf
    Ketone: negative   rare RBCs
    Bilirubin: negative   rare RBC and granular casts

    The student is upset with these results, but his instructor is not.

    a. Which opinion would you support?
    b. How could you prove your opinion?
    c. Explain the significance of each abnormal result.

29. As supervisor of the urinalysis laboratory, you are reviewing reports sent out by a new employee, and several results concern you. Tell what questions you would ask the person in each of the following cases.

    a. pH 7.0 with uric acid crystals
    b. 4 + glucose on a preoperative patient
    c. specific gravity 1.040
    d. yellow, hazy, negative blood, and many RBCs

30. The expected reading for glucose on your control sample is 3 + ; however, this morning it reads only 1 + . List in order the steps you would take to resolve this discrepancy.

6

Special Urinalysis Screening Tests

LEARNING OBJECTIVES

Upon completion of this chapter, the reader will be able to

1. explain the abnormal accumulation of metabolites in the urine in terms of overflow and renal disorders
2. name the metabolic defect in phenylketonuria and describe the clinical manifestations it produces
3. discuss the performance of the Guthrie and ferric chloride tests and their roles in the detection and management of phenylketonuria
4. list two tests used to screen for urinary tyrosine and its metabolites
5. name the abnormal urinary substance present in alkaptonuria and tell how its presence may be suspected
6. describe the appearance of urine containing excess melanin and two screening tests to detect its presence
7. describe a basic laboratory observation that has relevance in maple syrup urine disease
8. differentiate between the presence of urinary indican due to intestinal disorders and Hartnup disease
9. state the significance of increased urinary 5-HIAA
10. discuss the instructions that must be given to patients prior to the collection of samples to be tested for 5-HIAA
11. differentiate between cystinuria and cystinosis, including the differences that are found during analysis of the urine and the disease processes
12. name the chemical screening test for cystine
13. explain the chemical screening test used to distinguish between cystine and homocystine
14. describe the basic pathway for the production of heme and tell the two stages affected by lead poisoning
15. describe the appearance of urine that contains increased porphyrins
16. name the porphyrins measured by the Ehrlich reaction and those detected by fluorescence under a Wood's lamp
17. define mucopolysaccharides and name three syndromes in which they are involved
18. list three screening tests for the detection of urinary mucopolysaccharides
19. explain the reason for performing tests for urinary reducing substances on all newborns

In the previous five chapters, we have discussed the role of urinalysis in providing initial diagnostic information concerning metabolic dysfunctions of both renal and nonrenal origin. Much of this information came from the results of the routine urinalysis performed in the urinalysis laboratory, and some came from the measurement of renal function, which is shared between the urinalysis, clinical chemistry, and nuclear medicine laboratories. Although urine, as an end product of body metabolism, contains most substances or their degradation products that are found in the body, the procedures for analysis of these compounds often require sophisticated methodology and equipment not found in the urinalysis laboratory. Therefore, the role of the urinalysis laboratory becomes one of performing screening tests, the qualitative results of which are then utilized by the physician to determine whether additional tests should be performed. Examples of this include the detection by routine urinalysis of conditions such as diabetes mellitus, liver disorders, glomerular or tubular damage, and urinary tract infection. Additional testing of not only urine but also blood, other body fluids, or tissue may then be necessary. The scope of this book is not to cover these additional procedures performed in other sections of the laboratory but, rather, to provide students with a thorough understanding of the tests performed within the urinalysis laboratory and their significance as a part of the total diagnostic evaluation.

Although urinalysis laboratories vary as to the extent to which they are equipped to perform specialized procedures, certain tests—again, primarily of a qualitative nature—are considered the responsibility of the urinalysis laboratory. As shown in Table 6–1, the need to perform additional tests may be detected by the observations of alert laboratory personnel during the performance of the routine analysis or from observations by nursing staff and patients of abnormal specimen color and odor. In other instances, clinical symptoms and family histories are the deciding factors, and many laboratories perform a standardized battery of metabolic screening tests on newborns.[3]

Figure 6–1 shows an example of a newborn screening system. Except for the creatinine determination and the high-voltage electrophoresis, all initial tests can fall into the realm of the urinalysis laboratory. Creatinine is measured to determine urine concentration. Repeat specimens can be collected on dilute samples to prevent false-negative results, and aliquots of concentrated specimens are diluted to 0.2 mg of creatinine to prevent false-positive spot tests.[2]

OVERFLOW VERSUS RENAL DISORDERS

The accumulation of abnormal metabolic substances in the urine may be due to a variety of causes; however, these can generally be grouped into two categories, termed the overflow type and the renal type. Overflow disorders are due to increased production of metabolites resulting from the disruption of a normal metabolic pathway, causing increased serum concentrations of substances that either override the reabsorption ability

TABLE 6–1. Abnormal Metabolic Constituents or Conditions Detected in the Routine Urinalysis

COLOR	ODOR	CRYSTALS
Homogentisic acid	Phenylketonuria	Cystine
Melanin	Maple syrup urine disease	Leucine
Indican		Tyrosine
Porphyrins		

SCREENING OF THE URINE FOR METABOLIC DISEASE

COMPONENTS AND SEQUENCES OF FOLLOW-UP OF POSITIVE FINDINGS

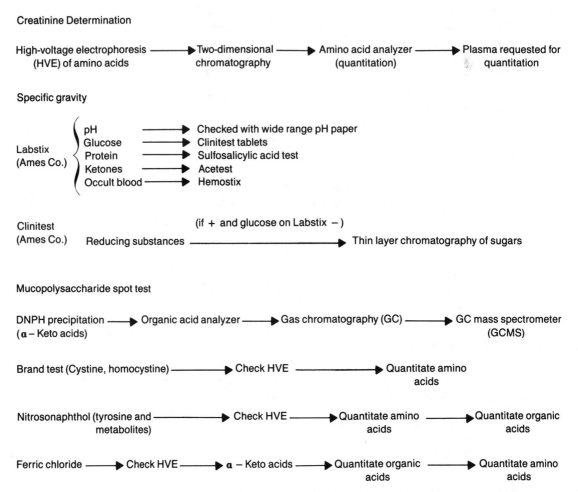

FIGURE 6–1. System of screening for metabolic disease. The components of the screen are shown at the left. Procedures employed to follow up positive findings are shown following the arrows toward the right. (From Bordon,[2] p 403, with permission.)

of the renal tubules or are not normally reabsorbed from the filtrate.[9] Abnormal accumulations of the renal type are due to malfunctions in the tubular reabsorption mechanism.

The most frequently encountered abnormalities are associated with metabolic disturbances that produce urinary overflow of substances involved in protein and carbohydrate metabolism. This is understandable when one considers the vast number of enzymes utilized in the metabolic pathways of proteins and carbohydrates and the fact that their function is essential to complete metabolism. Disruption of enzyme function can be caused by failure to inherit the gene to produce a particular enzyme, referred to as an "inborn error of metabolism,"[13] or by organ malfunction from disease or toxic reactions. Table 6–2 summarizes the most frequently encountered abnormal urinary metabolites and classifies their appearance according to functional defect. This table also includes those substances and conditions that are covered in this chapter.

TABLE 6–2. Major Disorders of Protein and Carbohydrate Metabolism Associated with Abnormal Urinary Constituents Classified as to Functional Defect

OVERFLOW		RENAL
INHERITED	METABOLIC	
Phenylketonuria	Tyrosinemia	Cystinuria
Tyrosinemia	Melanuria	Cystinosis
Alkaptonuria	Indican	
Maple syrup urine disease	5-Hydroxyindoleacetic acid	
Porphyria	Porphyria	
Mucopolysaccharidoses		
Melituria (galactosuria)		

AMINO ACID DISORDERS

PHENYLALANINE-TYROSINE METABOLISM

Many of the most frequently requested special urinalysis procedures are associated with the phenylalanine-tyrosine metabolic pathway. Major inherited disorders include phenylketonuria, tyrosyluria, alkaptonuria, and metabolic defects producing excessive amounts of melanin. The relationship of these varied disorders is illustrated in Figure 6–2.

Phenylketonuria

The most well-known of the aminoacidurias, phenylketonuria is estimated to occur in 1 of every 10,000 to 20,000 births and, if undetected, results in severe mental retardation. It was first identified in Norway by Ivan Folling in 1934, when a mother with other mentally retarded children reported a peculiar mousy odor to her child's urine.[33] Analysis of the urine showed increased amounts of the keto acids, including phenylpyruvate. As shown in Figure 6–2, this will occur when the normal conversion of phenylalanine to tyrosine is disrupted. Interruption of the pathway also produces children with fair complexions even in dark-skinned families, owing to the decreased production of tyrosine and its pigmentation metabolite, melanin.

Phenylketonuria (PKU) is caused by failure to inherit the gene to produce the enzyme phenylalanine hydroxylase. The gene is inherited as an autosomal recessive trait with no noticeable characteristics or defects exhibited by heterozygous carriers. Fortunately, screening tests are available for early detection of the abnormality, and most states have laws that require the screening of all newborns. Once discovered, dietary changes that eliminate phenylalanine, a major constituent of milk, from the infant's diet can prevent the excessive buildup of serum phenylalanine and can thereby avoid damage to the mental capabilities. As the child matures, alternate pathways of phenylalanine metabolism develop, and dietary restrictions can be eased. Many products, such as aspartamine, that contain large amounts of phenylalanine now have warnings for phenylketonuric persons.

The initial screening for PKU does not come under the auspices of the urinalysis laboratory, as increased blood levels of phenylalanine must, of course, occur prior to the

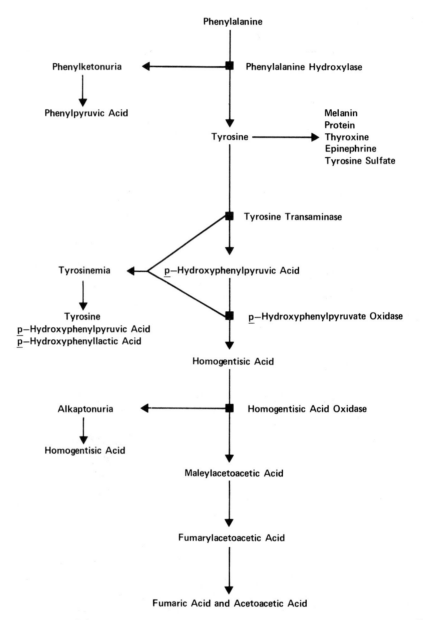

FIGURE 6–2. Phenylalanine and tyrosine metabolism. (Adapted from Frimpton,[12] and Kretchmer and Etzwiler.[23])

urinary excretion of phenylpyruvic acid, which may take from 2 to 6 weeks. Blood samples are usually obtained before the newborn is discharged from the hospital. To prevent false-negative results, care must be taken to ensure that there has been adequate ingestion of phenylalanine prior to collection of the sample, and tests should be repeated during an early visit to the pediatrician. More girls than boys escape detection of PKU during early tests because of slower rises in blood phenylalanine levels.[12] Urine testing can be used as a follow-up procedure in questionable diagnostic cases, as a screening test to ensure proper dietary control in previously diagnosed cases, and more recently, as a means of monitoring the dietary intake of pregnant women known to lack phenylalanine hydroxylase.[33]

The most well-known blood test for PKU is the bacterial inhibition test developed by Guthrie.[14] In this procedure, blood from a heelstick is absorbed into filter paper cir-

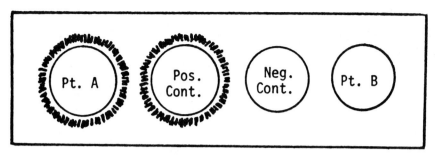

FIGURE 6–3. Guthrie's test.

cles. The blood-impregnated disks are then placed on culture media streaked with the organism *Bacillus subtilis*. If increased phenylalanine is present in the blood, it will counteract the action of an inhibitor of *Bacillus subtilis* that is present in the media, and growth will be observed around the paper disks. Notice that in Figure 6–3 the bacterial growth around the disk from Patient A corresponds to the positive control, indicating an increased level of phenylalanine. Modifications of the Guthrie test also will detect maple syrup urine disease, homocystinuria, tyrosinemia, histidinemia, valinemia, and galactosemia.[37] Several methods are available for measuring serum levels of phenylalanine, including an automated technique that measures the fluorescence of phenylalanine when it is heated in the presence of ninhydrin and L-leucyl-L-alanine or glycyl-L-leucine.[20]

Urine tests for phenylpyruvic acid are based upon the ferric chloride reaction performed either by tube or reagent strip (Phenistix, Ames Company, Elkhart, IN). As will be seen in other discussions in this chapter, the ferric chloride test is a nonspecific reaction and will react with many other amino acids and commonly ingested medications (see Table 6–3 later in chapter). This is particularly true when the tube test is used, inasmuch as more substances produce positive—although sometimes transient—reactions. Some brands of disposable diapers also produce false-positive reactions for PKU when tested with ferric chloride.[21] More consistent results are obtained using Phenistix, because the testing area contains a buffer to maintain an acid pH and magnesium ions to reduce the interference produced by urinary phosphates.[38] Phenistix produces a permanent blue-gray to green-gray color when a positive sample is tested. Comparison of results between ferric chloride tube tests and the Phenistix test sometimes can provide useful information in the screening for metabolic disorders.[22]

Tyrosyluria

The accumulation of excess tyrosine in the serum producing urinary overflow may be due to several causes and is not well categorized. As can be seen in Table 6–2, disorders of tyrosine metabolism may result from either inherited or metabolic defects. Also, because two reactions are directly involved in the metabolism of tyrosine, the urine may contain excess tyrosine or its degradation products, *p*-hydroxyphenylpyruvic acid and *p*-hydroxyphenyllactic acid. Most frequently seen is a transitory tyrosinemia in premature infants, which is caused by underdevelopment of the liver function necessary to complete the tyrosine metabolism.[32] This condition seldom results in permanent damage, but it may be confused with PKU when urinary screening tests are performed on newborns, because the ferric chloride test will produce a green color. However, this reaction can be distinguished from the PKU reaction with ferric chloride because the green color fades rapidly. Acquired severe liver disease also will produce tyrosyluria resembling that of the transitory newborn variety and, of course, is a more serious condition. In both instances, rarely seen tyrosine and leucine crystals may be observed during microscopic examination of the urine sediment. Hereditary disorders in which enzymes required in the metabolic pathway are not produced present a serious and usually fatal condition that results in both liver and renal disease and in the appearance of a generalized aminoaciduria.[23]

The recommended urinary screening tests for tyrosine and its metabolites are the nitroso-naphthol test and the Millon test. Like the ferric chloride test, the nitroso-naphthol test test is nonspecific and, as shown in Table 6–3, will react with compounds other than tyrosine and its metabolites. However, the presence of an orange-red color shows a positive reaction and indicates that further testing is needed. Millon's test will produce a red color in the presence of tyrosine or p-hydroxyphenylpyruvic acid. But because Millon's reagent contains the toxic substance mercury, the test is seldom performed in the routine clinical laboratory.

Alkaptonuria

Alkaptonuria was one of the six original "inborn errors of metabolism" described by Garrod in 1902. The name alkaptonuria was derived from the observation that urine from patients with this condition darkens after becoming alkaline from standing at room temperature. Therefore, the term "alkali lover," or alkaptonuria, was adopted. This metabolic defect is actually the third major one in the phenylalanine-tyrosine pathway and occurs from failure to inherit the gene to produce the enzyme homogentisic acid oxidase. Without this enzyme, the phenylalanine-tyrosine pathway cannot proceed to completion, and homogentisic acid accumulates in the blood, tissues, and urine. This condition does not usually manifest itself clinically in early childhood. But in later life, brown pigment becomes deposited in the body tissues and may eventually lead to arthritis.[10] A high percentage of persons with alkaptonuria develop liver and cardiac disorders.[36]

Homogentisic acid will react in several of the routinely used screening tests for metabolic disorders, including the ferric chloride test, in which a transient deep-blue color is produced in the tube test and a negative reaction occurs with Phenistix.[21] A yellow precipitate is produced in the Benedict's test or Clinitest, indicating the presence of a reducing substance. A more specific screening test for urinary homogentisic acid is to add alkali to freshly voided urine and to observe for darkening of the color; however, large amounts of ascorbic acid will interfere with this reaction.[37] The addition of silver nitrate and ammonium hydroxide also will produce a black urine. A spectrophotometric method to obtain quantitative measurements of both urine and plasma homogentisic acid is also available.[34]

Melanuria

We have been discussing the major phenylalanine-tyrosine metabolic pathway illustrated in Figure 6–2; however, as is the case with many amino acids, a second metabolic pathway also exists for tyrosine. This pathway is responsible for production of melanin, thyroxine, epinephrine, protein, and tyrosine-sulfate.[23] Of these substances, the major concern of the urinalysis laboratory is melanin, the pigment responsible for the color of hair, skin, and eyes. Deficient production of melanin results in albinism.

Like homogentisic acid, increased urinary melanin will produce a darkening of urine. The darkening appears after the urine is exposed to air. Elevation of urinary melanin is a serious finding that indicates the overproliferation of the normal melanin-producing cells (malignant melanoma). These tumors secrete a colorless precursor of melanin, 5,6-dihydroxyindole, which oxidizes to melanogen and then to melanin, producing the characteristic dark urine. Differentiation between the presence of melanin and homogentisic acid must certainly be made.

Melanin will react with ferric chloride, sodium nitroprusside (nitroferricyanide), and Ehrlich's reagent.[1] In the ferric chloride tube test, a gray or black precipitate will form in the presence of melanin and is easily differentiated from the transient blue-green color produced by homogentisic acid. The sodium nitroprusside test provides an additional screening test for melanin. A red color is produced by the reaction of melanin and sodium nitroprusside. Interference due to red color from acetone and creatinine can be avoided by adding glacial acetic acid, which will cause melanin to revert to a green-black color, whereas acetone turns purple, and creatinine becomes amber.[4]

SUMMARY OF URINE SCREENING TESTS FOR DISORDERS OF THE PHENYLALANINE-TYROSINE PATHWAY

Phenylketonuria
1. Phenistix
2. Ferric chloride tube test

Tyrosyluria
1. Nitroso-naphthol test
2. Millon's test

Alkaptonuria
1. Ferric chloride tube test
2. Benedict's test or Clinitest
3. Alkalization of fresh urine

Melanuria
1. Ferric chloride tube test
2. Sodium nitroprusside test
3. Ehrlich's test

MAPLE SYRUP URINE DISEASE

Although this is a rare disease, a brief discussion is included in this chapter because the urinalysis laboratory can provide valuable information for the essential early detection of this disease.

Maple syrup urine disease is referred to as a disorder of the branched chain amino acids produced by an inborn error of metabolism, inherited as an autosomal recessive trait. The amino acids involved are leucine, isoleucine, and valine. The metabolic pathway begins normally, with the transamination of the three amino acids in the liver to the keto acids α-ketoisovaleric, α-ketoisocaproic, and α-keto-β-methylvaleric. However, failure to inherit the gene for the enzyme necessary to produce oxidative decarboxylation of these keto acids results in their accumulation in the blood and urine.[9]

Newborns with maple syrup urine disease begin to exhibit clinical symptoms associated with failure to thrive after approximately 1 week. The presence of the disease may be suspected from these clinical symptoms; however, many other conditions have similar symptoms. Due to the rapid accumulation of keto acids in the urine, the disease may be detected by personnel in the urinalysis laboratory or in the nursery through the observation of a specimen that produces a strong odor resembling maple syrup. Even though a report of urine odor is not a part of the routine urinalysis, notifying the physician about this unusual finding can prevent the development of severe mental retardation and even death. Current studies have shown that if maple syrup urine disease is detected by the 11th day, the disorder can be controlled by dietary regulation and careful monitoring of urinary keto acid concentrations.[6]

The screening test most frequently performed for keto acids is the 2,4-dinitrophenyl-hydrazine (DNPH) reaction. Addition of DNPH to urine that contains keto acids will produce a yellow turbidity or precipitate. The DNPH test can also be used for home monitoring of diagnosed cases. Large doses of ampicillin will interfere with the DNPH reaction, and, as would be expected, the ferric chloride test will also be positive. Like many other urinary screening tests, the DNPH reaction is not specific for maple syrup urine disease, inasmuch as keto acids are present in other disorders, including phenylketonuria. Specimens with a positive reagent strip test for ketones will also produce a positive result. However, treatment can be started on the basis of odor, clinical symptoms, and a positive DNPH test while confirmatory procedures using amino acid chromatography are being performed. Studies also have shown that heterozygote carriers of the defective gene can be detected using the leukocyte decarboxylase test.[5]

TRYPTOPHAN METABOLISM DISORDERS

The major concern of the urinalysis laboratory in the metabolism of tryptophan is the increased urinary excretion of the metabolites indican and 5-hydroxyindoleacetic acid (5-HIAA). Figure 6–4 shows a simplified diagram of the metabolic pathways by which these substances are produced. Other metabolic pathways of tryptophan are not included because they do not relate directly to the urinalysis laboratory.

INDICAN

Under normal conditions, most of the tryptophan that enters the intestine is either reabsorbed for use by the body in the production of protein or is converted to indole by the intestinal bacteria and excreted in the feces.[27] However, in certain intestinal disorders (including obstruction; the presence of abnormal bacteria; malabsorption syndromes; and a rare inherited disorder, Hartnup disease) increased amounts of tryptophan are converted to indole. The excess indole is then reabsorbed from the intestine into the blood stream and circulated to the liver, where it is converted to indican and then excreted in the urine. Indican excreted in the urine is colorless until oxidized by exposure to air to form the dye indigo blue. Early diagnosis of Hartnup disease is sometimes made when mothers report a blue staining of their infant's diapers, referred to as the "blue diaper syndrome."[7] Urinary indican will react with acidic ferric chloride to form a deep-blue or violet color that can subsequently be extracted into chloroform.[4]

Except in cases of Hartnup disease, correction of the underlying intestinal disorder will return urinary indican levels to normal. The inherited defect in Hartnup disease affects not only the intestinal reabsorption of tryptophan but also the renal tubular reabsorption of other amino acids, resulting in a generalized aminoaciduria. The defective renal transport of amino acids does not appear to affect other renal tubular functions. Therefore, with proper dietary supplements, persons with Hartnup disease have a good prognosis.[19]

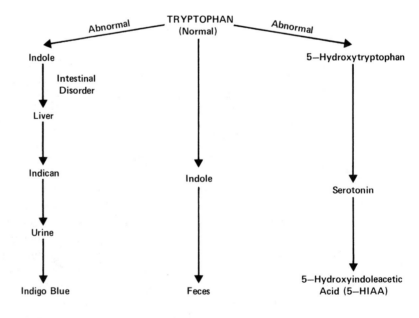

FIGURE 6–4. Tryptophan metabolism. (Adapted from Meister.[27])

5-Hydroxyindoleacetic Acid

As shown in Figure 6–4, a second metabolic pathway of tryptophan is for the production of serotonin utilized in the stimulation of smooth muscles. Serotonin is produced from tryptophan by the argentaffin cells in the intestine and is carried through the body primarily by the platelets. Normally, most of the serotonin is used by the body; only small amounts of its degradation product, 5-hydroxyindoleacetic acid (5-HIAA), are available for excretion in the urine. However, when malignant tumors involving the argentaffin cells develop, excess amounts of serotonin are produced, resulting in the elevation of urinary 5-HIAA levels.

The addition of nitrous acid and 1-nitroso-2-naphthol to urine that contains 5-HIAA causes the appearance of a purple to black color, depending on the amount of 5-HIAA present. The normal daily excretion of 5-HIAA is 2 to 8 mg, and argentaffin cell tumors will produce from 160 to 628 mg per 24 hours.[36] Therefore, the test is usually performed on a random or first morning specimen because there can be little chance of false-negative results. If a 24-hour sample is used, it must be preserved with hydrochloric or boric acid. Patients must be given explicit dietary instructions prior to the collection of any sample to be tested for 5-HIAA, because serotonin is a major constituent of foods such as bananas, pineapples, and tomatoes. Interference will also be caused by medications, including phenothiazines and acetanilids.[36] Patients should be requested to withhold medications for 72 hours prior to specimen collection.

CYSTINE METABOLISM DISORDERS

There are two distinct disorders of cystine metabolism that exhibit renal manifestations. Confusion as to their relationship existed for many years following the discovery by Wollaston in 1810 of renal calculi consisting of cystine.[17] It is now known that although both disorders are inherited, one is a defect in the renal tubular transport of amino acids (cystinuria) and the other is an inborn error of metabolism (cystinosis).

Cystinuria

As the name implies, the condition is characterized by elevated amounts of the amino acid cystine in the urine. The presence of increased urinary cystine is not due to a defect in the metabolism of cystine but, rather, to the inability of the renal tubules to reabsorb cystine filtered by the glomerulus. The demonstration that not only cystine but also lysine, arginine, and ornithine are not reabsorbed has ruled out the possibility of an error in metabolism even though the condition is inherited.[29] The disorder has two modes of inheritance: one in which reabsorption of all four amino acids—cystine, lysine, arginine, and ornithine—is affected, and the other condition, in which only cystine and lysine are not reabsorbed. The primary clinical consideration in cystinuria is the tendency of persons with defective reabsorption of all four amino acids to form calculi. Approximately 65 percent of these people can be expected to produce calculi early in life.[17]

Because cystine is much less soluble than the other three amino acids, laboratory screening determinations are based on the observation of cystine crystals in the sediment of concentrated or first morning specimens. Cystine is also the only amino acid found during the analysis of calculi from these patients. Elevations in the other three amino acids must be determined separately using chromatography procedures. A chemical screening test for urinary cystine can be performed using cyanide-nitroprusside. Reduction of cystine by sodium cyanide followed by the addition of nitroprusside will produce a red-purple color in a specimen that contains excess cystine. False-positive reactions will occur in the presence of ketones and homocystine, and additional tests that are specific for these substances may have to be performed to rule them out.

CYSTINOSIS

Regarded as a genuine inborn error of metabolism, cystinosis can occur in three variations, ranging from a severe fatal disorder developed in infancy to a benign form appearing in adulthood. The incomplete metabolism of cystine results in crystalline deposits of cystine in many areas of the body, including the cornea, bone marrow, lymph nodes, and internal organs. A major defect in the renal tubular reabsorption mechanism, referred to as the Fanconi syndrome, also occurs. Patients exhibit the inability to reabsorb amino acids, phosphorus, potassium, sugars, and water. Routine laboratory findings include polyuria, generalized aminoaciduria, positive tests for reducing substances, and lack of urinary concentration. In severe cases, there is a gradual progression to total renal failure.[29] Renal transplants and the use of cystine-depleting medications to prevent the buildup of cystine in other tissues are extending lives.

HOMOCYSTINURIA

Defects in the metabolism of homocystine can result in failure to thrive, cataracts, mental retardation, thromboembolic problems, and death. As mentioned earlier, increased urinary homocystine gives a positive result with the cyanide-nitroprusside test. Therefore, laboratory screening for homocystinuria can be performed by following a positive cyanide-nitroprusside test with a silver-nitroprusside test, in which only homocystine will react. The use of silver nitrate in place of sodium cyanide will reduce homocystine to its nitroprusside-reactive form but will not reduce cystine. Consequently, a positive reaction in the silver-nitroprusside test confirms the presence of homocystinuria.[38]

PORPHYRIN DISORDERS

Porphyrins are the intermediate compounds in the production of heme. The basic pathway for heme synthesis is illustrated in Figure 6–5. As can be seen, there are a number of stages at which production can be disrupted. The major disorders of porphyrin metabolism and the sites at which they interrupt the pathway are also shown in Figure 6–5.[28] Blockage of a pathway reaction will result in an accumulation of the product formed just prior to the interruption. Detection and identification of this compound in the urine serves as an aid to the diagnosis of the particular disorder. Conditions that result in the appearance of porphyrinuria are collectively termed porphyrias and can be inherited as inborn errors of metabolism or acquired through erythrocytic and hepatic malfunctions caused either by metabolic disease or exposure to toxic agents. Lead poisoning is the most common cause of porphyrinuria. The individual porphyrias will not be discussed separately in this section, and many varieties other than those shown in Figure 6–5 also exist.[8] Diagnosis of these other types often requires analysis of feces and erythrocytes; whereas the porphyrias shown in Figure 6–5 are more closely associated with the analysis of urine.

A possible indication of the presence of porphyrinuria is the observation of a red or port-wine color to the urine. However, porphobilinogen is excreted as a colorless compound, and the color change will not occur unless the urine is acidic and remains exposed to air for several hours. As we have seen with other inherited disorders, the presence of congenital porphyria is sometimes suspected from a red discoloration of an infant's diapers.[40]

The two screening tests for porphyrinuria utilize the Ehrlich reaction and fluorescence under ultraviolet light from a Wood's lamp. The Ehrlich reaction can be used only for the detection of aminolevulinic acid (ALA) and porphobilinogen; the fluorescent technique must be used for the other porphyrins. The Ehrlich reaction, including the Watson-Schwartz test for differentiation between the presence of urobilinogen and porphobilinogen, was discussed in detail in chapter 4. A more rapid method for the detection of in-

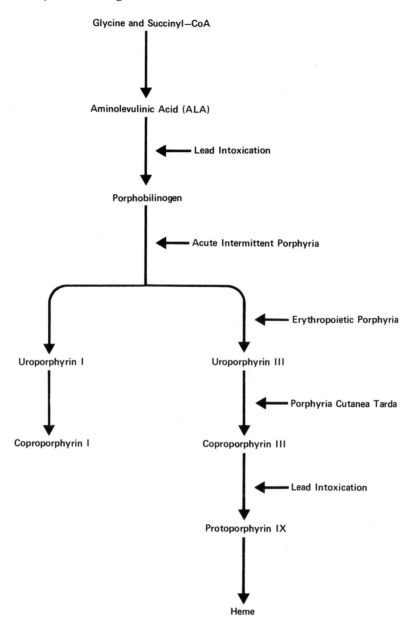

Glycine and Succinyl–CoA

Aminolevulinic Acid (ALA)

Lead Intoxication

Porphobilinogen

Acute Intermittent Porphyria

Erythropoietic Porphyria

Uroporphyrin I   Uroporphyrin III

Porphyria Cutanea Tarda

Coproporphyrin I   Coproporphyrin III

Lead Intoxication

Protoporphyrin IX

Heme

FIGURE 6–5. Pathway of heme formation, including stages affected by the major disorders of porphyrin metabolism. (Adapted from Miale.[28])

creased porphobilinogen that does not require a separation phase is the Hoesch test. It is most valuable for patients suspected of having acute attacks of porphyria and is performed by adding only 2 drops of urine to 1 or 2 milliliters of Ehrlich's reagent and observing for the appearance of a red color at the top of the solution.[24] When using the Ehrlich reaction to measure increased ALA, acetylacetone must be added to the specimen to convert the ALA to porphobilinogen prior to performing the Ehrlich test.[25] The detection of increased levels of urinary ALA is a primary screening test for lead poisoning. Mass screening programs often supply cation exchange paper dipsticks for the collection of specimens. The dipstick is allowed to dry and is mailed to the laboratory, where the ALA is eluted from the paper and tested.[16]

Fluorescent screening for the other porphyrins requires their extraction into a mixture of glacial acetic acid and ethyl acetate. The solvent layer is then examined under a Wood's lamp. Negative reactions have a faint blue fluorescence. Positive reactions will fluoresce as pink, violet, or red, depending upon the concentration of porphyrins. If the presence of interfering substances is suspected, the organic layer can be removed to a separate tube and 0.5 ml of hydrochloric acid added to the tube. Only porphyrins will be extracted into the acid layer, which will then produce a bright orange-red fluorescence. The fluorescence method will not distinguish among uroporphyrin, coproporphyrin, and protoporphyrin unless specimens are subjected to changes in pH, but it will rule out porphobilinogen and aminolevulinic acid.[15] The identification of the specific porphyrins requires additional extraction techniques and the analysis of fecal and erythrocyte samples.

SUMMARY OF PORPHYRIN SCREENING TESTS

Ehrlich's Reaction

1. Aminolevulinic acid
2. Porphobilinogen

Ultraviolet Light

1. Uroporphyrin
2. Coproporphyrin
3. Protoporphyrin

MUCOPOLYSACCHARIDE DISORDERS

Mucopolysaccharides, or glycosaminoglycans, are a group of large compounds located primarily in the connective tissue. They consist of a protein core with numerous polysaccharide branches. Inherited disorders in the metabolism of these compounds prevent the complete breakdown of the polysaccharide portion of the compounds, resulting in accumulation of the incompletely metabolized polysaccharide portions in the lysosomes of the connective tissue cells and their increased excretion in the urine.[38] The products most frequently found in the urine are dermatan sulfate, keratan sulfate, and heparan sulfate, with the appearance of a particular substance being determined by the specific metabolic error that was inherited. Therefore, identification of the specific degradation product present may be necessary to establish a specific diagnosis.[26] There are many types of mucopolysaccharidoses, but the best-known are Hurler's syndrome, Hunter's syndrome, and Sanfilippo's syndrome. In both Hurler's and Hunter's syndromes, the skeletal structure is abnormal and there is severe mental retardation; in Hurler's syndrome, mucopolysaccharides accumulate in the cornea of the eye. Both syndromes are usually fatal during childhood, whereas in Sanfilippo's syndrome, the only abnormality is mental retardation.[39]

Urinary screening tests for mucopolysaccharides are requested either as part of a routine battery of tests performed on all newborns or on infants who exhibit symptoms of mental retardation or failure to thrive. The most frequently used screening tests are the acid-albumin and cetyltrimethylammonium bromide (CTAB) turbidity tests and the metachromatic staining spot tests. In both the acid-albumin and the CTAB tests, a thick, white turbidity will form when these reagents are added to urine that contains mucopolysaccharides. Turbidity is usually graded on a scale of 0 to 4 after 10 minutes with acid-albumin and after 30 minutes with CTAB. Metachromatic staining procedures use basic dyes to react with the acidic mucopolysaccharides. MPS papers (Ames Company, Elkhart, IN) contain azure A dye, and urine that contains mucopolysaccharides will produce a blue spot that cannot be washed away by a dilute acidified methanol solution.[11] Papers also can be prepared by dipping Whatman no. 1 filter paper into a 0.59 percent azure A dye in 2 percent acetic acid and letting it air dry.[2]

OTHER SCREENING TESTS

COPPER REDUCTION TESTS

Discussed previously in chapter 4, the Benedict's and Clinitest copper reduction tests are included again in this section because they are usually included in newborn screening programs. The presence of increased urinary sugar (melituria) is most frequently due to an inherited disorder. In fact, pentosuria was one of Garrod's original six inborn errors of metabolism.[13] Fortunately, the majority of meliturias cause no disturbance to body metabolism.[18] However, the presence of galactosuria and fructosuria can have serious consequences. Therefore, when a positive test for urinary reducing substances is encountered with a negative reagent strip test for glucose, the specimen should be tested by thin-layer chromatography for the identification of these sugars.

Screening for fructose can be done by boiling 5 ml of urine with 5 ml of 25 percent hydrochloric acid for 5 minutes, adding 5 mg of resorcinol, boiling 10 seconds, and observing for a red precipitate. Confirmation of the presence of fructose is made if the precipitate will dissolve in ethanol and produce a red color.[55]

SULKOWITCH'S TEST

Historically, the Sulkowitch test was used as a qualitative measurement of urinary calcium. Sulkowitch's reagent (which contains oxalic acid, ammonium oxalate, and glacial acetic acid) reacts with urinary calcium, creating turbidity due to the precipitation of calcium oxalate. Turbidity is graded on a scale of 0 to 4. It is now accepted that a qualitative measurement of urinary calcium provides little useful diagnostic information, and urinary calcium in conjunction with serum calcium is quantitatively measured in the chemistry laboratory.

SUMMARY

A summary of urinary screening tests is presented in Table 6–3.

TABLE 6–3. Summary of Urinary Screening Tests[2, 22, 31, 38]

TEST	DISORDER	OBSERVATION
Color	Homogentisic acid	Black
	Melanuria	Black
	Indicanuria	Dark blue
	Porphyrinuria	Port wine
Odor	Phenylketonuria	Mousy
	Maple syrup urine disease	Maple syrup
	Cystinuria	Sulfur
	Cystinosis	Sulfur
	Homocystinuria	Sulfur
Crystals	Tyrosyluria	Sheaths of fine needles
	Cystinuria	Colorless hexagonal plates

(continued)

TABLE 6–3. *Continued*

TEST	DISORDER	OBSERVATION
Ferric chloride tube test Slowly add 5 drops of 10 percent ferric chloride to 1 ml of urine.	Phenylketonuria Tyrosyluria Homogentisic acid Melanuria Maple syrup urine disease Indicanuria 5-HIAA	Blue-green Transient green Transient blue Gray-black Green-brown Violet-blue with chloroform Blue-green
Phenistix	Phenylketonuria Tyrosyluria	Gray-green Transient green
Nitroso-naphthol To 5 drops of urine in a spot plate, add 1 ml of 2.63 N nitric acid, 1 drop of 2.5 percent sodium nitrite and 0.1 ml 1-nitroso-2-napthol. Mix. Observe in 5 minutes.	Phenylketonuria Tyrosyluria Maple syrup urine disease 5-HIAA	Red Red Red Violet with nitric acid
2,4-Dinitrophenylhydrazine (DNPH) Add 1 ml of 0.2 percent 2,4-DPNH in 2M HCl to 1 ml urine. Observe for ppt. in 5 minutes.	Phenylketonuria Tyrosyluria Maple syrup urine disease	Yellow Yellow Yellow
Cyanide-nitroprusside To 1 ml of urine in a spot plate, add 2 drops concentrated NH_4OH followed by 0.5 ml 5 percent sodium cyanide. In 10 minutes add 5 drops sodium nitroprusside. Observe color.	Cystinuria Cystinosis Homocystinuria	Red-purple Red-purple Red-purple
Silver-nitroprusside To 1 ml of urine in a spot plate, add 2 drops concentrated NH_4OH followed by 0.5 ml 5 percent silver nitrate. In 10 minutes add 5 drops sodium nitroprusside. Observe color.	Homocystinuria	Red-purple

TABLE 6–3. *Continued*

TEST	DISORDER	OBSERVATION
Ehrlich's reaction Add 2 drops urine to 1 to 2 ml Ehrlich's reagent. Observe color at top.	Porphyrinuria Melanuria	Red Red
Acid-albumin turbidity test	Mucopolysaccharidoses	White turbidity
Cetyltrimethylammonium bromide (CTAB)	Mucopolysaccharidoses	White turbidity
MPS paper Spot 1 drop of urine on dry MPS paper. Dry. Wash 5 minutes (in 1 ml acetic acid + 200 ml methanol diluted to a liter). Dry. Observe for blue spot.	Mucopolysaccharidoses	Blue spot
Reducing substances	Homogentisic acid Cystinosis Melituria	Orange-red Orange-red Orange-red

REFERENCES

1. Beeler, MF and Henry, JB: Melanogenuria: Evaluation of several commonly used laboratory procedures. JAMA 176:52–54, 1961.
2. Bordon, M: Screening for metabolic disease. In Nyhan, WL: Abnormalities in Amino Acid Metabolism in Clinical Medicine. Appleton-Century-Crofts, Norwalk, CT, 1984.
3. Bradley, GM: Urinary screening tests in the infant and young child. Hum Pathol 2(2):309–320, 1971.
4. Bradley, M and Schumann, GB: Examination of the urine. In Henry, JB (ed): Clinical Diagnosis and Management of Laboratory Methods. WB Saunders, Philadelphia, 1984.
5. Chuang, DT, et al: Detection of heterozygotes in MSUD: Measurement of branched-chain α-ketoacid dehydrogenase and its components in cell cultures. Am J Hum Genet 34(3):416–424, 1982.
6. Clow, CL, Reade, TH, and Scriver, CR: Outcome of early and long-term management of classical maple syrup urine disease. Pediatrics 68(6):856–862, 1981.
7. Drummond, KN, et al: The blue diaper syndrome: Familial hypercalcemia. Am J Med 37:928–948, 1964.
8. Eades, L: The porphyrins and porphyrias. Annu Rev Med 12:251–270, 1961.
9. Effron, ML: Aminoaciduria. N Engl J Med 272:1058–1067, 1965.
10. Flanagen, SM: Urinalysis problem. Am J Med Technol 48(5):375–376, 1982.
11. Free, AH and Free, HM: Urodynamics: Concepts Relating to Routine Urine Chemistry. Ames Co, Division of Miles Laboratories, Elkhart, Indiana, 1978.
12. Frimpton, GW: Aminoacidurias due to inherited disorders of metabolism. N Engl J Med 1289:835–901, 1973.

13. Garrod, AE: Inborn Errors of Metabolism. Henry Froude & Hodder & Stoughton, London, 1923.

14. Guthrie, R: Blood screening for phenylketonuria. JAMA 178(8):863, 1961.

15. Haining, RG, Hulse, T, and Labbe, RF: Rapid porphyrin screening of urine, stool and blood. Clin Chem 16(6):460–466, 1961.

16. Hankin, L., et al: Simplified method for mass screening for lead poisoning based on α-aminolevulinic acid in urine. Clin Pediatr 9:707, 1970.

17. Harris, H and Robson, EB: Cystinuria. Am J Med 22:774–783, 1957.

18. Hiatt, HH: Pentosuria. In Stanbury, JB, Wyngaarden, JB, and Fredrickson, DE (eds): The Metabolic Basis of Inherited Diseases. McGraw-Hill, New York, 1983.

19. Jepson, JB: Hartnup's disease. In Stanbury, JB, Wyngaarden, JB, and Fredrickson, DS (eds): The Metabolic Basis of Inherited Diseases. McGraw-Hill, New York, 1983.

20. Kirkman, H, et al: Fifteen year experience with screening for phenylketonuria with an automated fluorometric method. Am J Hum Genet 34(5):743–752, 1982.

21. Kishel, M and Lighty, P: Some diaper brands give false-positive tests for PKU. N Engl J Med 300(4):200, 1979.

22. Knight, JA and Wu, JT: Screening profile for detection of inherited metabolic disorders. Laboratory Medicine 13(11):681–687, 1982.

23. Kretchmer, N and Etzwiler, DD: Disorders associated with the metabolism of phenylalanine and tyrosine. Pediatrics 21:445–475, 1958.

24. Lamon, J, With, TK, and Redeker, AG: The Hoesch test: Bedside screening for urinary porphobilinogen in patients with suspected porphyria. Clin Chem 20:1438–1440, 1974.

25. Mauzerall, D and Granick, S: The occurrence and determination of D-amino-levulinic acid and porphobilinogen in urine. J Biol Chem 219:435–436, 1956.

26. McKusick, VA, and Neufeld, EF: The mucopolysaccharide storage diseases. In Stanbury, JB, Wyngaarden, JB, and Fredrickson, DS (eds): The Metabolic Basis of Inherited Diseases. McGraw-Hill, New York, 1983.

27. Meister, A: Biochemistry of the Amino Acids. Academic Press, New York, 1965.

28. Miale, JB: Laboratory Medicine: Hematology. CV Mosby, St. Louis, 1982.

29. Nyahn, WL: Abnormalities in Amino Acid Metabolism in Clinical Medicine. Appleton-Century-Crofts, Norwalk, CT, 1984.

30. Pankau, EF: Purple urine bags. J Urol 130(2):372–373, 1983.

31. Perry, TL, Hansen, SH, and MacDougall, L: Urinary screening tests in the prevention of mental deficiency. Can Med Assoc J 95:89–97, 1966.

32. Race, GJ and White, MG: Basic Urinalysis. Harper & Row, Hagerstown, Maryland, 1979.

33. Ragsdale, N and Koch, R: Phenylketonuria: Detection and therapy. Am J Nurs 64:90–96, 1964.

34. Seegmiller, JE, et al: An enzymatic spectrophotometric method for the determination of homogentisic acid in plasma and urine. J Biol Chem 236:774–777, 1961.

35. Seliwanoff, S: Ber Deutch. Chem Gesellsch, 20:181, 1887. In Essential Fructosuria. Report of Three Cases with Metabolic Studies (S. Silberg and M. Reiner, eds) Arch Intern Med, 54:412, 1934.

36. Sjoerdsma, A, Weissbach, H, and Udenfriend, S: Simple test for diagnosis of metastatic carcinoid (argentaffinoma). JAMA 159(4):397, 1955.

37. Stanbury, JB: The Metabolic Basis of Inherited Diseases. McGraw-Hill, New York, 1983.

38. Thomas, GH and Howell, RR: Selected Screening Tests for Metabolic Diseases. Yearbook Medical Publishers, Chicago, 1973.

39. Thompson, JS and Thompson, MW: Genetics in Medicine. WB Saunders, Philadelphia, 1978.

40. Waldenstrom, J: The porphyrias as inborn errors of metabolism. Am J Med 22:758–773, 1957.

STUDY QUESTIONS (Choose one best answer)

1. The appearance of abnormal metabolites in the urine due to a defect categorized as an "overflow type" may be caused by all of the following except
   a. inborn errors of metabolism
   b. serum concentrations exceeding the tubular reabsorption
   c. abnormalities in the tubular reabsorption mechanism
   d. disruption of normal enzyme function by exposure to toxic substances

2. Phenylketonuria is caused by
   a. excessive ingestion of milk products containing phenylalanine
   b. inability to metabolize tyrosine
   c. lack of the enzyme phenylalanine hydroxylase
   d. a mousy odor in the urine

3. Initial screening for PKU performed on newborns prior to their discharge from the hospital utilizes a blood sample rather than a urine sample because
   a. urine samples are more difficult to collect
   b. blood is routinely collected on all newborns for other tests
   c. it is easier to measure phenylalanine than phenylpyruvic acid
   d. increased serum phenylalanine occurs earlier than increased urine phenylpyruvic acid

4. The Guthrie test is
   a. a bacterial inhibition test
   b. a fluorometric procedure
   c. a chemical procedure measured by spectrophotometer
   d. a bacterial agglutination test

5. Detection of urine phenylpyruvic acid by Phenistix utilizes a chemical reaction between phenylpyruvic acid and
   a. sodium chloride
   b. ferric chloride
   c. phenylalanine
   d. *Bacillus subtilis*

6. The color of a positive PKU reaction on Phenistix is
   a. yellow-orange
   b. red-orange
   c. gray-green
   d. brown-black

7. A transient positive reaction on Phenistix may indicate
   a. deterioration of the test strip
   b. reduced levels of phenylpyruvic acid
   c. the presence of phenylalanine
   d. tyrosine and its metabolites

8. The abnormal metabolite that is present in the urine in alkaptonuria is
   a. homogentisic acid
   b. alkaptonpyruvate
   c. phenylpyruvate
   d. tyrosine

9. A routine urinalysis is performed on a specimen that has turned dark after standing in the laboratory. The urine is acidic and has negative chemical tests except for the appearance of a red color on the ketone area of the reagent strip. One should suspect

    a. phenylketonuria
    b. diabetic ketosis
    c. alkaptonuria
    d. melanuria

10. Although urine odor is not included in the routine urinalysis, it can be important in the early detection of

    a. branched chain amino acid disorders
    b. straight chain amino acid disorders
    c. all amino acid disorders
    d. no medically important amino acid disorders

11. Confirmation of maple syrup urine disease is made on the basis of

    a. urine odor
    b. positive 2,4-dinitrophenylhydrazine test
    c. positive ferric chloride test
    d. amino acid chromatography

12. Analysis of urine from an infant whose mother reported a blue staining on the diapers showed increased levels of indican and a generalized aminoaciduria. On the basis of these findings, the infant was diagnosed as having

    a. an intestinal obstruction
    b. a protein malabsorption syndrome
    c. Fanconi's syndrome
    d. Hartnup disease

13. Under normal conditions, tryptophan that is not reabsorbed in the intestine is removed from the body as

    a. indican in the urine
    b. indole in the liver
    c. indole in the feces
    d. serotonin in the urine

14. The finding of increased amounts of the serotonin degradation product 5-hydroxy-indoleacetic acid in the urine is indicative of

    a. platelet disorders
    b. intestinal obstruction
    c. malabsorption syndromes
    d. argentaffin cell tumors

15. Interference will occur in 5-HIAA tests if patients are not properly instructed in

    a. specimen collection procedures
    b. dietary restrictions
    c. time of specimen collection
    d. coordination of blood and urine samples

16. Place the appropriate letter in front of the statement that best matches the condition:

    a. cystinuria   b. cystinosis
    ____ true inborn error of metabolism
    ____ defective reabsorption of cystine, lysine, ornithine, and arginine
    ____ tendency to form renal calculi
    ____ Fanconi's syndrome
    ____ generalized aminoaciduria

17. Chemical screening tests for cystine will produce false-positive results in the presence of urinary ketones because
    a. cystine is not reduced by sodium cyanide
    b. cystine should be tested using only chromatography
    c. the test reagent is nitroprusside
    d. glucose present in diabetic ketosis concentrates the specimen

18. Porphyrins are intermediary compounds in the formation of
    a. amino acids
    b. serotonin
    c. heme
    d. bilirubin

19. The presence of porphobilinogen in the urine can be suspected when
    a. acidic urine turns a port-wine color after standing
    b. alkaline urine turns a port-wine color after standing
    c. freshly excreted urine is acidic and port wine in color
    d. freshly excreted urine is alkaline and port wine in color

20. Urine from a child suspected of having lead poisoning has a red fluorescence under a Wood's lamp. This finding is
    a. inconsistent with lead poisoning because aminolevulinic acid does not fluoresce
    b. consistent with lead poisoning because coproporphyrin fluoresces under ultraviolet light
    c. consistent with lead poisoning only if uroporphyrin is also increased
    d. consistent only if protoporphyrin can be demonstrated using Ehrlich's reagent

21. Hurler's and Sanfilippo's syndromes present with mental retardation and increased urinary
    a. porphyrins
    b. amino acids
    c. maltose
    d. mucopolysaccharides

22. The presence of urinary reducing substances is of particular concern in
    a. pregnant women
    b. newborns
    c. adolescent males
    d. menopausal women

23. The Sulkowitch test screens for urinary
    a. glucose
    b. oxalate
    c. calcium
    d. ammonia

CASE STUDIES

1. During a 2-week vacation in Hawaii, Tom Richardson develops stomach pains. Immediately upon his return, he visits his physician, who orders a chemistry profile, urine-5-HIAA, and an upper GI series. All tests are normal except the 5-HIAA, and Mr. Richardson's stomach discomfort has ended.

    a. What could account for the elevated 5-HIAA?
    b. How can Tom's physician verify that he does not have a tumor of the argentaffin cells?

2. Bobby Williams, age 8, is admitted through the emergency department with a ruptured appendix. Although surgery is successful, Bobby's recovery is slow, and the physicians are concerned about his health prior to the ruptured appendix. Bobby's mother states that he has always been noticeably underweight despite a balanced diet and strong appetite and that his younger brother exhibits similar characteristics. A note in his chart from the first postoperative day reports that the evening nurse noticed a purple coloration on the urinary catheter bag.[30]

   a. Is the catheter bag color significant?
   b. What additional tests should be run?
   c. What condition can be suspected from this history?
   d. What is Bobby's prognosis?

3. Baby girl Miller receives the customary PKU test prior to her discharge from the hospital, and the result is negative. At her 6-week examination, the physican observes that she is lethargic and has failed to thrive. He orders a battery of metabolic screening tests. The ferric chloride tube test turns a gray-green-brown color, and a yellow-white precipitate forms with 2,4-dinitrophenylhydrazine. Negative reactions are found with cyanide-nitroprusside, MPS paper, and Clinitest.

   a. What two conditions do these results suggest?
   b. What further testing could be done?
   c. Is the negative PKU test of any significance? Explain your answer.

CEREBROSPINAL FLUID

LEARNING OBJECTIVES

Upon completion of this chapter, the reader will be able to

1. list the three major functions of cerebrospinal fluid (CSF)
2. distribute CSF specimen tubes numbered 1, 2, and 3 to their appropriate laboratory sections
3. describe the appearance of normal and infectious CSF
4. define xanthochromia and state its significance
5. differentiate between the appearance of a blood specimen caused by a cerebral hemorrhage and one that resulted from a traumatic spinal tap
6. calculate CSF white and red blood cell counts when given the number of cells seen, amount of specimen dilution, and the squares counted in the Neubauer chamber
7. briefly explain the methods used to correct for white blood cells and protein that are artificially introduced during a traumatic tap
8. name the type of white blood cell primarily associated with bacterial, viral, tubercular, and parasitic meningitis
9. describe and give the significance of abnormal macrophages in the CSF
10. give two differences in the appearance of normal choroidal cells and malignant cells
11. identify and state the significance of abnormal cells in the CSF
12. state the normal value for CSF total protein
13. list three pathologic conditions that produce an elevated CSF protein
14. discuss the basic principles associated with the turbidimetric and the dye-binding methods of CSF protein analysis
15. state the normal CSF glucose value
16. name the possible pathologic significance of a decreased CSF glucose
17. briefly discuss the diagnostic value of CSF lactate, glutamine, and lactic dehydrogenase determinations
18. name the microorganism associated with a positive India ink preparation
19. state the diagnostic value of the Limulus Lysate test
20. determine whether a suspected case of meningitis is most probably of bacterial, viral, fungal, or tubercular origin, when presented with pertinent laboratory data

FORMATION AND PHYSIOLOGY

First recognized by Cotugno in 1764, cerebrospinal fluid (CSF) is the third major fluid of the body.[16] The CSF provides a physiologic system to supply nutrients to the nervous

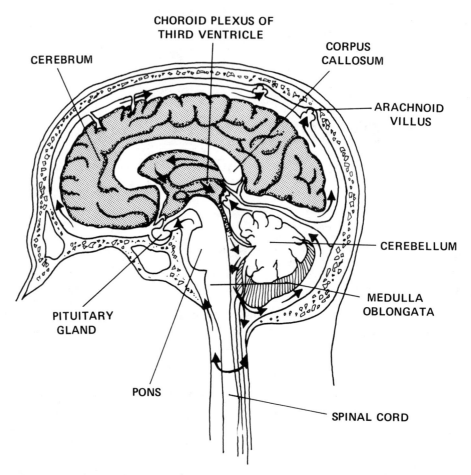

CHOROID PLEXUS OF
THIRD VENTRICLE

CEREBRUM

CORPUS
CALLOSUM

ARACHNOID
VILLUS

CEREBELLUM

MEDULLA
OBLONGATA

PITUITARY
GLAND

PONS

SPINAL CORD

FIGURE 7–1. The flow of cerebrospinal fluid through the brain and spinal column.

tissue, to move metabolic wastes, and to produce a mechanical barrier to cushion the brain and spinal cord against trauma. Approximately 20 ml of fluid are produced every hour in the choroid plexuses and reabsorbed by the arachnoid villi to maintain a total volume of 140 to 170 ml in adults, and 10 to 60 ml in neonates.[27,36] Figure 7–1 depicts the flow of the CSF through the brain and spinal column. Production of CSF in the choroid plexuses is by filtration under hydrostatic pressure across the choroidal capillary wall and active transport secretion by the choroidal epithelial cells. Tightly fitting junctions between the endothelial cells of the capillaries and the choroid plexuses restrict entry of macromolecules such as protein, insoluble lipids, and substances bound to serum proteins. The chemical composition of the fluid does not resemble an ultrafiltrate of plasma due to bidirectional active transport between the CSF, interstitial brain fluid, brain cells, and blood in the brain capillaries. The term blood-brain barrier is used to represent all of the bidirectional exchanges between the blood, CSF, and brain, replacing the older individual terms CSF-blood barrier, CSF-brain barrier, and blood-brain barrier.[11]

SPECIMEN COLLECTION

Cerebrospinal fluid is routinely collected by lumbar puncture between the third, fourth, or fifth lumbar vertebrae. Although this is not a complicated procedure, it does require certain precautions, including measurement of the intracranial pressure and careful technique to prevent the introduction of infection or the damaging of neural tissue. Speci-

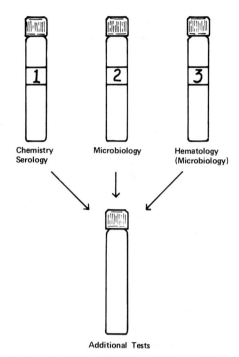

FIGURE 7–2. Cerebrospinal fluid specimen collection tubes.

mens are usually collected in three sterile tubes, labeled 1, 2, and 3 in the order in which they are withdrawn. Tube 1 is used for chemical and serologic tests; tube 2 is used for microbiology; tube 3 is used for the cell count, because it is the least likely to contain cells introduced by the spinal tap procedure. If possible, a fourth tube may be drawn for microbiology inasmuch as it is less likely to contain skin contaminants. Supernatant fluid that is left over after each section has performed its tests may be used for additional chemical or serologic tests. Excess fluid should not be discarded until there is no further use for it (Fig. 7–2). Specimens for additional chemical and serologic tests should be frozen. Hematology tubes are refrigerated, and microbiology tubes remain at room temperature.

CEREBROSPINAL FLUID IN THE HEMATOLOGY LABORATORY

APPEARANCE

The initial appearance of the normally crystal clear CSF can provide valuable diagnostic information (Table 7–1). Examination of the fluid occurs first at the bedside and is also included in the hematology report. The major terminology used to describe CSF appearance includes crystal clear, cloudy or turbid, milky, xanthochromic, and bloody. A cloudy, turbid, or milky specimen can be the result of an increased protein or lipid concentration, but it also may be indicative of infection, with the cloudiness being caused by the presence of white blood cells. All specimens should be treated with extreme care because they can be highly contagious, and gloves are always worn.

Xanthochromia is a term used to describe CSF supernatant that is either pink, orange, or yellow. A variety of factors can cause the appearance of xanthochromia, with the most common being the presence of red blood cell degradation products. Depending on the amount of blood and the length of time it has been present, the color will vary

TABLE 7–1. Clinical Significance of CSF Appearance

APPEARANCE	CAUSE	MAJOR SIGNIFICANCE
Crystal clear		Normal
Hazy, turbid, cloudy, smoky, milky	WBCs	Meningitis
	RBCs	Hemorrhage
		Traumatic tap
	Microorganisms	Meningitis
	Protein	Disorders that affect blood-brain barrier
		Production of IgG within CNS
Oily	Radiographic contrast material	
Bloody	RBCs	Hemorrhage
Xanthochromic	Hemoglobin	Old hemorrhage
		Lysed cells from traumatic tap
	Bilirubin	RBC breakdown
		Elevated serum bilirubin
	Merthiolate	Contamination
	Carotene	Increased serum levels
	Protein	SEE ABOVE
Clotted	Protein	SEE ABOVE
	Clotting factors	Introduced by traumatic tap
Pellicle formation	Protein	Tubercular meningitis
	Clotting factors	

from pink (very slight amount of oxyhemoglobin) to orange (heavy hemolysis) to yellow (conversion of oxyhemoglobin to unconjugated bilirubin). Other causes of xanthochromia include elevated serum bilirubin, presence of the pigment carotene, markedly increased protein concentrations, and melanoma pigment. Xanthochromia that is due to immature liver function is also commonly seen in infants, particularly in those who are premature.

TRAUMATIC COLLECTION

Grossly bloody CSF can be an indication of intracranial hemorrhage, but it also may be due to the puncture of a blood vessel during the spinal tap procedure. Three visual examinations of the collected specimens can usually determine whether the blood is the result of hemorrhage or "traumatic tap."

1. **Uneven Distribution of Blood.** Blood from a cerebral hemorrhage will be evenly distributed throughout the three CSF specimen tubes; whereas a traumatic tap will have the heaviest concentration of blood in tube 1, with gradually diminishing amounts in tubes 2 and 3. Streaks of blood also may be seen in specimens acquired following a traumatic procedure.

2. **Clot Formation.** Fluid collected from a traumatic tap may form clots due to the introduction of plasma fibrinogen into the specimen. Bloody CSF caused by intracranial hemorrhage will not contain enough fibrinogen to clot. Diseases in which damage to the blood-brain barrier allows increased filtration of protein and coagulation factors will also cause clot formation but do not usually produce a bloody fluid. These conditions include meningitis, Froin's syndrome, and

blockage of CSF circulation through the subarachnoid space. A classic weblike pellicle is associated with tubercular meningitis and is frequently seen after overnight refrigeration of the fluid.[31]

3. **Xanthochromic Supernatant.** Red blood cells must usually remain in the CSF for approximately 2 hours before hemolysis begins; therefore, a xanthochromic supernatant would be the result of blood that has been present longer than that introduced by the traumatic tap. Care should be taken, however, to consider this examination in conjunction with those previously discussed, because a very recent hemorrhage would produce a clear supernatant, and introduction of serum protein from a traumatic tap could also cause the fluid to appear xanthochromic. Microscopic examination of the fluid for the presence of crenated red blood cells, once considered an additional confirmation that blood was the result of intracranial hemorrhage, is not a reliable indication of hemorrhage and should not be used.[26]

CELL COUNT

The cell count that is routinely performed on CSF specimens is the leukocyte (WBC) count. As discussed earlier, the presence and significance of red blood cells can usually be ascertained from the appearance of the specimen. Therefore, red blood cell counts are usually performed only when a traumatic tap has occurred and it is necessary to correct for the leukocytes or protein introduced into the specimen. Any cell count should be performed immediately, because white blood cells (particularly granulocytes) and red blood cells will begin to lyse within an hour, with 40 percent of the leukocytes disintegrating after 2 hours.[2,14] Specimens that cannot be analyzed immediately should be refrigerated.

Methodology

Normal adult CSF contains 0 to 5 white blood cells per microliter. The number is higher in children, and as many as 30 mononuclear cells per microliter can be considered normal in newborns.[22] Specimens that contain up to 200 white blood cells or 400 red blood cells per microliter may appear clear, so it is necessary to examine all specimens microscopically.[13] Electronic counters cannot be used for CSF because of the variations in background counts and the possibility of falsely elevating normal or moderately high counts. An improved Neubauer counting chamber (Fig. 7–3) is routinely used.

The standard Neubauer calculation formula used for blood cell counts is also applied to CSF cell counts to determine the number of cells per μl. This is

$$\frac{\text{Number of cells counted} \times \text{dilution}}{\text{Number of squares counted} \times \text{volume of 1 square}} = \text{cells/}\mu\text{l}$$

This formula can be used for both diluted and undiluted specimens and offers flexibility in the number and size of the squares counted. Many varied calculations are available, including condensations of the formula to provide single factors by which to multiply the cell count. Keep in mind that the purpose of any calculation is to convert the number of cells counted in a specific amount of fluid to the number of cells that would be present in one microliter of fluid. Therefore, a factor can be used only when the dilution and counting area are specific for that factor.

The methodology presented in this chapter eliminates the need to correct for the volume counted by counting the four large corner squares (0.4 μl) and the large center square (0.1 μl).[43]

Example:

$$\text{Number of cells counted} \times \text{dilution} \times \frac{1\ \mu\text{l}}{1\ \mu\text{l}\ (0.1 \times 10)\ \text{counted}} = \text{cells/}\mu\text{l}$$

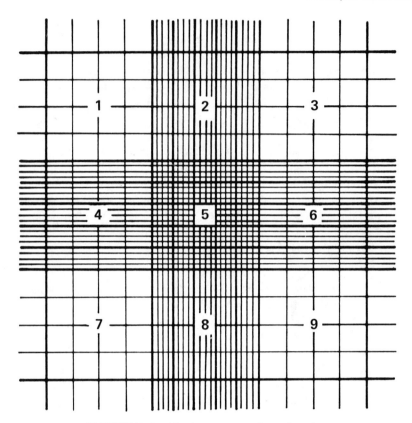

FIGURE 7–3. Neubauer counting chamber.

Total Cell Count

Clear specimens may be counted undiluted, provided no overlapping of cells is seen during the microscopic examination. Dilutions have historically been made using Thoma pipettes and aspirators. To avoid the dangers of mouth-pipetting, the following method using calibrated automatic pipettes is recommended.[43]

CLARITY	DILUTION	AMOUNT OF SAMPLE	AMOUNT OF DILUENT
Sl. Hazy	1:10	30 μl	270 μl
Hazy	1:20	30 μl	570 μl
Sl. Cloudy	1:100	30 μl	2970 μl
Sl. Bloody			
Cloudy	1:200	30 μl	5970 μl
Bloody			
Turbid	1:10,000	0.1 ml of a 1:100 dilution	9.9 ml

Dilutions for total cell counts are made with normal saline, mixed by inversion, and loaded into the hemocytometer with a Pasteur pipette. Cells are counted in the four corner squares and the center square on both sides of the hemocytometer. The number of cells counted multiplied by the dilution factor equals the number of cells per microliter.

White Blood Cell Count

Lysis of red blood cells must be obtained prior to performing the white blood cell count on either diluted or undiluted specimens. Specimens requiring dilution can be diluted in the manner described above, substituting 3 percent acetic acid or a toluidine blue O and saponin solution that lyses the red blood cells and stains the white cells.[21] To prepare a clear specimen for counting, place 4 drops of mixed specimen in a clean tube. Rinse a Pasteur pipette with glacial acetic acid, draining thoroughly, and draw the 4 drops of CSF into the rinsed pipette. Allow the pipette to sit for 1 minute, mix the solution in the pipette, discard the first drop, and load the hemocytometer.

As in the total cell count, cells are counted in the four corner squares and the center square on both sides of the hemocytometer and the number is multiplied by the dilution factor to obtain the number of white blood cells per microliter. If a lesser number of squares are counted, the standard Neubauer formula should be used to obtain the number of cells per microliter.

Recent studies have shown good correlation between the Multistix leukocyte esterase test and the presence of white blood cells in the CSF. However, this is recommended as a screening test and not to replace the actual count.[25]

Red Blood Cell Count

The total cell count per microliter minus the white blood cell count per microliter equals the red blood count per microliter.

Corrections for Contamination

Calculations are possible to correct for white blood cells and protein artificially introduced into the CSF as the result of a traumatic tap. Determination of the CSF red blood cell count and the blood red and white cell counts is necessary to perform the correction. By determining the ratio of WBCs to RBCs in the peripheral blood and comparing this ratio with the number of contaminating RBCs, the number of artificially added WBCs can be calculated using the formula.[22]

$$WBC\ (added) = \frac{WBC\ (blood) \times RBC\ (CSF)}{RBC\ (blood)}$$

A true CSF white blood cell count can then be obtained by subtracting the "added" WBCs from the actual count. When peripheral blood RBC and WBC counts are in the normal range, many laboratories choose to simply subtract either 1 or 2 cells for every 1200 RBCs, or 1 cell for every 750 RBCs present in the CSF.[38] Studies have shown that the corrected WBC count is often lower than would be expected, indicating that correction of bloody fluids may be of little value in determining the need to culture.[33,34]

Differential Count

Specimen Preparation. Once CSF has been found to contain cells, identifying the type or types of cells present is a valuable diagnostic aid. The differential count should be performed on a stained smear and not from the cells in the counting chamber. Poor visualization of the cells as they appear in the counting chamber has led to a common laboratory practice of reporting only the percentage of mononucluear and polynuclear cells present. To ensure that the maximum number of cells are available for examination, the specimen should be concentrated prior to the preparation of the smear. Methods available for specimen concentration include filtration, sedimentation, cytocentrifugation, and ordinary centrifugation. Most laboratories that do not have a cytocentrifuge concentrate specimens with ordinary centrifugation. The specimen is centrifuged for 5 to 10 minutes; supernatant fluid is removed and saved for additional tests; slides made from the suspended sediment are allowed to air-dry and are stained with Wright's stain. When performing the differential count, 100 cells should be counted, classified, and reported in terms of percentage. If the cell count is low and it is not possible to find 100 cells, report only the numbers of the cell types seen. An advantage to the filtration, sedimentation, and cytocentrifugation techniques is that they produce better cell yields.

As little as 0.2 ml of CSF combined with one drop of 30 percent albumin produces an adequate cell yield when processed with the cytocentrifuge. Addition of albumin increases the cell yield and decreases cellular distortion frequently seen on cytocentrifuged

TABLE 7–2. Cytocentrifuge Recovery Chart[43]

NUMBER OF WBC COUNTED IN CHAMBER	NUMBER OF CELLS COUNTED ON CYTOCENTRIFUGE SLIDE
0	0–40
1–5	20–100
6–10	60–150
11–20	150–250
20	250

specimens. Cellular distortion may include cytoplasmic vacuoles and processes, nuclear clefting, prominent nucleoli, and cellular clumping resembling malignancy. Cells from both the center and periphery of the slide should be examined because cellular characteristics may vary between areas of the slide. A daily control slide for bacteria should also be prepared using 0.2 ml saline and 2 drops of 30 percent albumin. The slide is stained and examined if bacteria are seen on a patient's slide.[43]

Table 7–2 provides a cytocentrifuge recovery chart for comparison with chamber counts. The chamber count should be repeated if too many cells are seen on the slide, and a new slide should be prepared if not enough cells are seen on the slide.[43]

Significance of Normal Cells. The cells found in normal CSF are primarily lymphocytes and monocytes. Adults usually have a predominance of lymphocytes to monocytes (70:30); whereas monocytes are more prevalent in children.[23] Improved concentration methods are also showing occasional neutrophils in normal CSF[21] **(Color Plates 49 and 50).** The presence of increased numbers of these normal cells (termed pleocytosis) is considered abnormal, as is the finding of immature leukocytes, eosinophils, plasma cells, macrophages, increased tissue cells, and malignant cells. The CSF differential count is most frequently associated with its role in providing diagnostic information about the type of microorganism that is causing an infection of the meninges (meningitis). A high CSF white cell count of which the majority of the cells are neutrophils is considered indicative of bacterial meningitis **(Color Plates 51, 52, and 64).** Likewise, a moderately elevated CSF white cell count with a high percentage of lymphocytes and monocytes suggests meningitis of viral, tubercular, fungal, or parasitic origin. A low cell count—below 25 cells per cubic milliliter—with increased mononuclear cells is indicative of multiple sclerosis.[39] With this preliminary laboratory information and clinical observations, the physician can begin treatment without having to wait for the microbiology reports.

Significance of Abnormal Cells. As can be seen from Table 7–3, many pathologic conditions other than meningitis can be associated with the finding of abnormal cells in the CSF. Therefore, laboratory personnel should be careful not to overlook other types of cells because they become so accustomed to finding neutrophils, lymphocytes, and monocytes. The same care that is applied to reporting the blood differential should be given the CSF differential, keeping in mind that an even larger variety of cells is found in the CSF. Cell forms differing from those found in blood include macrophages, choroid plexus and ependymal cells, and malignant cells. Macrophages **(Color Plate 53)** appear within 2 to 4 hours after the introduction of red blood cells into the fluid and are frequently seen following repeated taps. The finding of increased macrophages containing red blood cells is indicative of a previous hemorrhage **(Color Plate 54).** The macrophages may also contain hemosiderin granules and hematoidin crystals **(Color Plates 55 to 58).**

Ependymal cells and choroid plexus cells **(Color Plates 59 to 60)** from the lining of the ventricles are not considered clinically significant. They are most frequently seen fol-

TABLE 7–3. Predominant Cells Seen in Cerebrospinal Fluid

TYPE OF CELL	MAJOR CLINICAL SIGNIFICANCE	MICROSCOPIC FINDINGS
Lymphocyte	Normal Viral, tubercular, and fungal meningitis Multiple sclerosis	All stages of development may be found
Neutrophil	Bacterial meningitis Early cases of viral, tubercular, or fungal meningitis Cerebral hemorrhage	Granules may be less prominent than in blood[20] Cells disintegrate rapidly
Monocyte	Chronic bacterial meningitis Viral, tubercular, and fungal meningitis Multiple sclerosis	Found mixed with lymphocytes and neutrophils
Eosinophil	Parasitic infections Allergic reactions Intracranial shunts (hydrocephalus)	Same appearance as seen in blood
Macrophages	Viral and tubercular meningitis RBCs in spinal fluid	May contain phagocytized RBCs appearing as empty vacuoles or ghost cells and hemosiderin granules
Pia arachnoid mesothelial (PAM) cells	Normal, mixed reactions, including neutropohils, lymphocytes, monocytes, and plasma cells	Resemble young monocytes with a round, not indented, nucleus[21]
Blast forms	Acute leukemia	Lymphoblasts or myeloblasts
Plasma cells	Multiple sclerosis Lymphocyte reactions	Transitional and classic forms seen
Ependymal cells Choroidal cells	Normal trauma Diagnostic procedures	Seen in clusters with distinct nuclei and distinct cell walls
Malignant cells	Metastatic carcinomas	Seen in clusters with fusing of cell borders and nuclei

lowing diagnostic procedures such as pneumoencephalography or in fluid obtained from ventricular taps or during neurosurgery.

Increased eosinophils (**Color Plate 61**) are seen in parasitic infections, reactions to foreign protein in the CSF, and intracranial shunt malfunctions.

Nucleated red blood cells (**Color Plate 62**) are seen as a result of bone marrow contamination during the spinal tap.

Plasma cells (**Color Plate 78**) and reactive lymphocytes (**Color Plate 63**) are seen in the CSF during viral infections and may be found in multiple sclerosis. A combination of transformed and normal cells is usually found.

A mixed reaction containing neutrophils, lymphocytes, monocytes, and pia arachnoid mesothelial cells is frequently found in viral, fungal, and tubercular meningitis and is also seen in the latter stages of bacterial meningitis. Intracellular and extracellular bacteria and budding yeast (**Color Plates 64 and 65**) may also be found on the differential smear.

The presence of blast forms and immature white blood cells is seen when there is CNS involvement in leukemias and lymphomas (**Color Plates 66 to 70**).

Metastatic carcinoma cells from many sources will appear in the CSF. They frequently appear in clusters and must be distinguished from normal clusters of ependymal, choroid plexus, and mesothelial cells (**Color Plates 59, 60, 71**). Fusing of cell walls and nuclear irregularities and hyperchromatic nucleoli are seen in clusters of malignant cells (**Color Plate 72**). Any suspicious slides should be referred to a pathologist.

CEREBROSPINAL FLUID IN THE CHEMISTRY LABORATORY

Because CSF is formed by filtration of the plasma, one would expect to find the same chemicals in the CSF as are found in the plasma. This is essentially true; however, because the filtration process is selective and the chemical composition is also adjusted by the blood-brain barrier, normal values for CSF chemicals are not the same as the plasma values. Abnormal values are the result of alterations in the permeability of the blood-brain barrier or increased production or metabolism by the neural cells in response to a pathologic condition, and they seldom have the same diagnostic significance as plasma abnormalities. The clinically important CSF chemicals are relative few in number, although under certain conditions, it may be necessary to measure a larger variety. Many CSF metabolites are currently being investigated in association with neurologic disorders and are discussed by Kjeldsberg and Knight.[21] We will concentrate on the most routinely requested analyses.

CEREBROSPINAL PROTEIN

Normal Protein Composition

The most frequently performed chemical test on CSF is the protein determination. Normal CSF contains a very small amount of protein. Normal values for total CSF protein are usually listed as 15 to 45 mg per dl, with slightly higher values found in infants and elderly people. Notice that this value is reported in milligram per deciliter and not grams per deciliter, as are plasma protein concentrations. In general, the CSF contains protein fractions similar to those found in serum; however, as can be seen in Table 7–4, the ratio of CSF proteins to serum proteins varies among the fractions. As in serum, albumin comprises the majority of CSF protein. But in contrast to serum, prealbumin is the second

TABLE 7–4. CSF and Serum Protein Correlations*

	CSF (mg/dl)	SERUM (mg/dl)	RATIO
Prealbumin	1.7	23.8	14
Albumin	15.5	3600	236
Ceruloplasmin	0.1	36.6	366
Transferrin	1.4	204	142
IgG	1.2	987	802
IgA	0.13	175	1346

*Adapted from Fishman.[11]

most prevalent fraction in CSF. The alpha globulins include primarily haptoglobin and ceruloplasmin. Transferrin is the major beta globulin present, although a separate carbohydrate-deficient transferrin fraction, referred to as "tau," is seen in CSF and not in serum. Cerebrospinal fluid gamma globulin is primarily IgG, with only a small amount of IgA. IgM, fibrinogen, and beta lipoprotein are not found in normal CSF.[11]

Clinical Significance of Elevated Protein

Elevated total protein values are most frequently seen in pathologic conditions, but abnormally low values will be present when fluid is leaking from the central nervous system. The causes of elevated CSF protein include damage to the blood-brain barrier, production of immunoglobulins within the central nervous system, decreased clearance of normal protein from the fluid, and degeneration of neural tissue. Meningitis and hemorrhage—conditions that result in damage to the blood-brain barrier—are the most common causes of elevated CSF protein. They, of course, are also associated with the production of cloudy fluids and increased cell counts. However, many other neurologic disorders can cause an elevation in the CSF protein, and it is not unusual to find an abnormal result on a clear fluid with a low cell count. Also, just as blood cells can be artificially introduced into a specimen by a traumatic tap, so can plasma protein. A correction calculation similar to that used in cell counts is available for protein measurements; however, if the correction is to be used, it is essential that both the cell count and the protein determination be done on the same tube.[13] When the blood hematocrit and serum protein values are normal, it is acceptable to subtract 1 mg per dl protein for every 1200 RBCs counted.[22]

Methodology

The two most routinely used techniques for measuring total CSF protein utilize the principles of turbidity production or dye-binding ability. Turbidimetric methods have been available for many years and rely on the precipitation of protein by either sulfosalicylic acid or trichloroacetic acid. The reagent of choice is trichloroacetic acid because it will precipitate both albumin and globulin equally. Unless sulfosalicylic acid is combined with sodium sulfate, albumin will contribute more to the turbidity than globulin. Standards should be prepared from human serum and not from albumin. The turbidimetric method using trichloroacetic acid has also been adapted to the Automated Chemistry Analyzer (ACA, Dupont Company, Wilmington, DE). Dye-binding techniques offer the advantages of smaller sample size and less interference from external sources. The recent development of dye-binding procedures that are almost as rapid and easy to perform as the turbidity methods has greatly increased their acceptance in laboratories. A convenient laboratory procedure is provided by the Microprotein Rapid Stat Kit (Pierce Chemical Company, Rockford, IL). This method utilizes the dye Coomassie brilliant blue G-250 and the principle of "protein error of indicators" discussed in chapter 4. Coomassie brilliant blue dye is used because it will bind to a variety of proteins rather than just to albumin. The color change of the pH-stabilized dye reagent from red to blue occurs when protein binds to the dye.[15] The concentration of protein present will determine the amount of blue color produced, thereby allowing a mathematical conversion of the intensity of the blue color present to the concentration of protein present (Beer's law).

Until recently, biuret used routinely for serum protein analysis had not been considered sensitive enough for CSF analysis. A modification of the biuret method that measures the rate of alkaline biuret-protein chelate formation rather than the colorimetric end-point reaction has been incorporated by the Astra (Automated Stat/Routine Analyzer, Beckman Instruments, Inc., Brea, CA). The method can accurately determine CSF protein concentrations between 12 and 750 mg per dl and correlates well with measurements on the Automated Chemistry Analyzer.[10]

Protein Fractions

Both the turbidimetric and the dye-binding techniques are designed to measure total protein concentration. However, diagnosis of neurologic disorders associated with abnormal

CSF protein often requires measurement of the individual protein fractions. Protein that appears in the CSF as a result of damage to the integrity of the blood-brain barrier will contain fractions proportional to those in plasma, with albumin present in the highest concentration. Diseases, including multiple sclerosis, that stimulate the immunocompetent cells in the central nervous system will show a higher proportion of IgG.[42]

To determine whether IgG is increased because it is being produced within the central nervous system or is only elevated due to increased serum levels, an IgG profile is performed. The profile consists of an IgG-to-albumin ratio and an IgG index. Because albumin is not produced within the central nervous system, increased IgG accompanied by increased albumin represents damage to the barrier, and the ratio will resemble that of normal CSF. In contrast, production of IgG within the central nervous system will raise the IgG-to-albumin ratio. Because variations in the serum albumin concentrations can affect the IgG-to-albumin ratio, a more precise evaluation can be made using the IgG index.[17] The formula for this index is[41]

$$\frac{\text{CSF IgG/serum IgG}}{\text{CSF albumin/serum albumin}}$$

By controlling for variations in serum albumin, actual synthesis of IgG within the central nervous system can be assessed. Normal volunteers have been shown to produce an index below 0.60, whereas a higher index is usually seen in multiple sclerosis.[35]

Techniques for the measurement of CSF albumin and globulin include electrophoresis, radial immunodiffusion, and nephelometry. Electrophoresis will provide an overall picture of all proteins present, whereas radial immunodiffusion and nephelometry measure individual fractions.

Electrophoresis

The recommended support medium for electrophoresis is agarose gel, and several commercial systems are available.[20] A characteristic oligoclonal banding can be seen on agarose gel in up to 95 percent of patients with multiple sclerosis.[7] Oligoclonal bands can be seen in other diseases of immune origin; however, in the majority of these cases, oligoclonal bands are also found on serum electrophoresis and represent specific antibodies.[5] In multiple sclerosis, banding is not seen in serum, and the bands are characteristic for each patient rather than a specific antibody. Immunofixation electrophoresis and isoelectric focusing techniques can also be used to detect oligoclonal banding and will demonstrate very small bands.[1]

Other procedures that are associated with the fractionation of CSF protein include serologic methods for the detection of myelin-based protein from the degradation of neural tissue, and two previously used tests, the Pandy and colloidal gold tests.

CEREBROSPINAL FLUID GLUCOSE

Glucose enters the CSF by selective transport across the blood-brain barrier, which results in a normal value that is approximately 60 to 70 percent that of the plasma glucose. If the plasma glucose is 100 mg per dl, then a normal CSF glucose would be approximately 65 mg per dl. For an accurate evaluation of CSF glucose, it is necessary to run a blood glucose test for comparison. The blood glucose should be drawn at least 30 minutes prior to the spinal tap to allow time for equilibration between the blood and fluid. Cerebrospinal fluid glucose is analyzed using the same procedures employed for blood glucose. Specimens should be tested immediately because glycolysis occurs rapidly in the CSF. As will be seen shortly, a decreased value due to in-vitro glycolysis could produce a serious error in patient treatment.

Clinical Significance. The diagnostic significance of CSF glucose is confined to the finding of values that are decreased in relation to plasma values. Elevated CSF glucose is always a result of plasma elevations. Low CSF glucose values can be of considerable diagnostic value in determining the causative agents in meningitis. The finding of a markedly decreased CSF glucose accompanied by an increased white cell count and a large percentage of neutrophils is most indicative of bacterial meningitis. If the white cells are lymphocytes instead of neutrophils, tubercular meningitis is suspected. Likewise, if a normal CSF glucose is found with an increased number of lymphocytes, the diagnosis would favor viral meningitis. Keep in mind that classic laboratory patterns such as those just described may not be found in all cases of meningitis, but they can be helpful when they are present.

Decreased CSF glucose values are thought to be caused primarily by alterations in the mechanisms of glucose transport across the blood-brain barrier and by increased utilization of glucose by the brain cells. Consumption of glucose by the microorganisms and leukocytes that are present in the fluid could not account for such decreased values, as it would not be possible to explain the variations in glucose concentrations seen in the different types of meningitis.[28]

CEREBROSPINAL FLUID LACTATE

The determination of CSF lactate levels is becoming a valuable aid in the diagnosis and management of meningitis cases. Enzymatic analysis can now be performed routinely in the clinical laboratory on automated analyzers. In bacterial, tubercular, and fungal meningitis, the elevation of CSF lactate to levels above 25 mg per dl occurs much more consistently than does the depression of glucose and provides the physician with more reliable information when the initial diagnosis is difficult.[3] Cerebrospinal fluid lactate levels remain elevated during initial treatment but fall rapidly when treatment is successful, thus offering a sensitive method for evaluating the effectiveness of antibiotic therapy.

Destruction of tissue within the central nervous system because of oxygen deprivation causes the production of increased CSF lactic acid levels. Therefore, elevated CSF lactate is not limited to meningitis and can result from any condition that decreases the flow of oxygen to the tissues.[37] Red blood cells contain high concentrations of lactate, and falsely elevated results may be obtained on xanthochromic fluid.[21]

CEREBROSPINAL FLUID GLUTAMINE

Another chemical test that is frequently performed on CSF and not on blood is the glutamine test. Glutamine is produced in the central nervous system by the brain cells from ammonia and α-ketoglutarate. This process serves to remove the toxic metabolic waste product ammonia from the central nervous system. The normal concentration of glutamine in the CSF is 8 to 18 mg per dl.[18] Elevated levels are found in association with liver disorders that result in increased blood and CSF ammonia. Increased synthesis of glutamine is caused by the excess ammonia that is present in the central nervous system; therefore, the determination of CSF glutamine provides an indirect test for the presence of excess ammonia in the CSF. Several methods of assaying glutamine are available and are based on the measurement of ammonia liberated from the glutamine.[12] This is preferred over the direct measurement of CSF ammonia because the concentration of glutamine remains more stable than that of the volatile ammonia in the collected specimen.[11] The CSF glutamine level also correlates with clinical symptoms much better than does the blood ammonia.[18]

As the concentration of ammonia in the CSF increases, the supply of α-ketoglutarate becomes depleted; glutamine can no longer be produced to remove the toxic ammonia, and coma ensues. Some disturbance of consciousness is almost always seen when glutamine levels are over 35 mg per dl. Therefore, the CSF glutamine test is a recommended procedure for all patients with coma of unknown origin. Requests for the test also have increased recently because 75 percent of children with Reye's syndrome have elevated CSF glutamine.[12]

CEREBROSPINAL LACTIC DEHYDROGENASE

Throughout the years, many enzymes in the CSF have been studied, but little clinical application of CSF enzyme tests has resulted. However, the development of techniques for separating and measuring the isoenzymes of lactic dehydrogenase has renewed interest in the CSF enzymes.[8] Lactic dehydrogenase can be separated into five isoenzymes, termed LD1, LD2, LD3, LD4, and LD5. The LD isoenzymes appear in the CSF following the destruction of particular cells, primarily neutrophils, lymphocytes, and brain cells. Brain tissue contains LD1 and LD2; lymphocytes contain LD2 and LD3; and neutrophils contain LD4 and LD5.[32] Therefore, LD isoenzymes can be utilized to confirm the presence of neutrophils and lymphocytes in the CSF, thereby aiding in the diagnosis of meningitis and, in cases of viral meningitis, providing an indication of the amount of tissue destruction that is occurring.

SUMMARY OF CSF CHEMISTRY TESTS

Protein

1. Normal concentration is 15 to 45 mg per dl.
2. Elevated values are most frequently seen in meningitis, hemorrhage, and multiple sclerosis.

Glucose

1. Normal value is 60 to 70 percent of the plasma concentration.
2. Decreased levels are seen with bacterial and tubercular meningitis.

Lactate

1. Levels above 25 mg per dl are found with bacterial, tubercular, and fungal meningitis.

Glutamine

1. Normal concentration is 8 to 18 mg per dl.
2. Levels above 35 mg per dl are associated with some disturbance of consciousness.

Lactic Dehydrogenase

1. Isoenzymes LD1 and LD2 are found in brain tissue.
2. Isoenzymes LD2 and LD3 are found in lymphocytes.
3. Isoenzymes LD4 and LD5 are found in neutrophils.

CEREBROSPINAL FLUID IN THE MICROBIOLOGY LABORATORY

The role of the microbiology laboratory in the analysis of CSF lies in the identification of the causative agent in meningitis. For positive identification, the microorganism must be recovered from the fluid by growing it on the appropriate culture medium. This can take anywhere from 24 hours in cases of bacterial meningitis to 6 weeks for tubercular meningitis. Consequently, in many instances, the CSF culture is actually a confirmatory rather than a diagnostic procedure. However, the microbiology laboratory does have several methods available to provide information for a preliminary diagnosis. These methods include the Gram stain, acid-fast stain, India ink preparation, Limulus Lysate test, counterimmunoelectrophoresis, and latex agglutination tests (Table 7–5).

GRAM STAIN

The Gram stain is routinely performed on CSF from all suspected cases of meningitis, although its value lies in the detection of bacterial and fungal organisms. All smears and cultures should be performed on concentrated specimens because often only a few or-

TABLE 7–5. Summary of the Major Laboratory Results for the Differential Diagnosis of Meningitis

BACTERIAL	VIRAL	TUBERCULAR	FUNGAL
Elevated WBC count	Elevated WBC count	Elevated WBC count	Elevated WBC count
Neutrophils present	Lymphocytes present	Lymphocytes and monocytes present	Lymphocytes and monocytes present
Marked protein elevation	Moderate protein elevation	Moderate to marked protein elevation	Moderate to marked protein elevation
Decreased glucose	Normal glucose	Decreased glucose	Normal to decreased glucose
Elevated lactate	Normal lactate	Elevated lactate	Elevated lactate
Elevated LD4 and LD5	Elevated LD2 and LD3		
Positive Limulus Lysate with gram-negative organisms		Pellicle formation	Positive India ink with *Cryptococcus neoformans*

ganisms are present at the onset of the disease. The CSF should be centrifuged at 1500 g for 15 minutes, and slides and cultures should be prepared from the sediment.[29] Even when concentrated specimens are used, there is at least a 10 percent chance that cultures will be negative. Thus, it is also recommended that blood cultures be taken, because the causative organism will often be present in both the CSF and the blood.[21] A CSF Gram stain is one of the most difficult slides to interpret because the number of organisms present is usually small and they can easily be overlooked, resulting in a false-negative report. Also, false-positive reports can occur if precipitated stain or debris is mistaken for microorganisms. Therefore, considerable care should be taken when interpreting a Gram stain.

Acid-fast or fluorescent antibody stains ae not routinely performed on specimens, unless tubercular meningitis is suspected. Considering the length of time required to culture mycobacteria, a positive report from this smear is extremely valuable. Specimens from possible cases of fungal meningitis are Gram stained, but they should also have an India ink preparation performed on them. The India ink preparation is designed to detect one of the most common causes of fungal meningitis, *Cryptococcus neoformans*. However, it is not as sensitive as the reverse latex agglutination tests.[40]

LIMULUS LYSATE TEST

The Limulus Lysate test is relatively new to the field of CSF analysis; it can be useful in the diagnosis of meningitis caused by gram-negative bacteria.[30] The reagent for this test is prepared from the blood cells of the horseshoe crab (*Limulus polyphemus*). These cells, termed amebocytes, contain a copper complex that gives them a blue color, thereby making the horseshoe crab a true "blue blood." Endotoxin found in the cell walls of gram-negative bacteria coagulates the amebocyte lysate within 1 hour if incubated at 37°C. The test is sensitive to minute amounts of endotoxin and will detect all gram-negative bacteria. The procedure must be performed using sterile technique to prevent false-positive results caused by contamination of specimens or tubes with endotoxin. Considerable amounts of endotoxin can be found in tap water.

IMMUNOLOGIC PROCEDURES

Counterimmunoelectrophoresis (CIE) is a serologic procedure utilized by the microbiology laboratory for detection and identification of bacterial antigens in the CSF. Although it is not as sensitive as the limulus lysate test, if positive, it provides rapid identification of the infectious organism.[9] Because not all bacteria possess the chemical characteristics needed for the reaction to take place, CIE is limited to the detection and identification of *Hemophilus influenzae, Streptococcus pneumoniae, Neisseria meningitidis, Escherichia coli,* and group B streptococci. Cross-over reactions, including one between *E. coli* and *H. influenzae,* may occur between these organisms.[9]

Recently developed latex agglutination and enzyme-linked immunosorbent assay (ELISA) methods do not require the specialized equipment needed for CIE and provide a more rapid means for detecting and identifying microorganisms in CSF. However, the Gram stain is still the recommended method for detection of organisms.[6]

CEREBROSPINAL FLUID IN THE SEROLOGY LABORATORY

Serologic examination of the CSF has historically been associated with the diagnosis of tertiary or neurosyphilis. The use of penicillin in the early stages of syphilis has greatly reduced the number of cases of neurosyphilis. Consequently, the number of requests for serologic tests for syphilis on CSF is lower. However, detection of the antibodies associated with syphilis in the CSF still remains a necessary diagnostic procedure. Although many different serologic tests for syphilis are available when testing blood, the recommended procedure for testing CSF is the VDRL (Venereal Disease Research Laboratories), which uses sensitized antigen and quantitation.[19] The fluorescent treponemal antibody absorption (FTA-ABS) test, although more sensitive than the VDRL, should not be used because contamination by even a minute amount of FTA-reactive blood may produce a positive CSF reaction.[6]

TEACHING CEREBROSPINAL FLUID ANALYSIS

Many of the problems that occur in the analysis of CSF are the result of inadequate training of the personnel performing the tests. This is understandable when one considers that not only is CSF difficult to collect there is often very little fluid left for student practice after the required tests have been run.

Preparation of simulated fluids by adding blood cells to saline has met with limited success due to the instability of the cells in saline and the inability to perform routine chemical analyses for glucose and protein. More satisfactory results can be achieved using the procedure described below, which provides the teaching laboratory with a specimen suitable for all types of cell analyses and glucose and protein determinations. The advantages of this simulated spinal fluid over others include the absence of bicarbonate, which may cause bubbling with acidic diluting fluids; the absence of calcium, which prevents clot formation when blood is added; stability for 48 hours under refrigeration; no distortion of cellular morphology; and the presence of glucose and protein.[24]

SIMULATED SPINAL FLUID (SSF) PROCEDURE*

EQUIPMENT AND REAGENTS

1. Whole blood is collected the same day in EDTA. The "ideal" blood specimen for preparing SSF has a white count around 10×10^9 per liter, a low platelet count, and a normal-appearing differential with at least 20 percent lymphocytes. Five to 7 ml of blood are needed to prepare 50 ml of SSF.
2. HBSS, Hanks' balanced salt solution (10x) without phenol red, sodium bicarbonate, calcium, or magnesium (Grand Island Biological Company, Grand Island, NY). Dilute 1:10 with deionized water.
3. Thirty percent bovine serum albumin (BSA).
4. Macrohematocrit tubes.
5. Capillary (Pasteur type) pipettes—both standard and 9-inch length.
6. Horizontal head centrifuge. A Beckman TJ6 model (Beckman Instruments, Inc., Palo Alto, CA) was used for this study.

PROCEDURE

1. For each SSF sample, dispense 50 ml diluted balanced salt solution into a 125-ml Erlenmeyer flask. (The amount of balanced salt solution may be varied; 50 ml will make approximately 30 aliquots of SSF.)
2. Centrifuge the blood in the original collection tube at $300 \times g$ for 5 minutes. A gray-pink buffy coat layer should be visible at the interface between the plasma and the red cells.
3. Aspirate off as much plasma as possible with a capillary pipette. Do not disturb the top (buffy coat) layer. Discard the plasma.
4. With a 9-inch capillary pipette and a circular motion, aspirate off the remaining plasma and the entire buffy coat layer. A small amount of the red cell layer will be aspirated into the pipette at the same time. This is acceptable.
5. Fill a macrohematocrit tube with this buffy coat mixture. Do not mix blood specimens from more than one source in one tube (they may agglutinate).
6. Centrifuge the macrohematocrit tube at $900 \times g$ for 10 minutes.
7. Pipette off as much of the plasma as possible and discard it. If a definite white layer (platelets) is visible above the gray buffy coat, carefully remove as much of it as possible without disturbing the gray layer.
8. Using a clean 9-inch capillary pipette, aspirate off the buffy coat (and as little of the red cell layer as possible) and add it to the flask containing diluted balanced salt solution. Rinse the pipette several times.
9. Mix well, and check the concentration of red cells and white cells by examining the SSF in a hemocytometer.
10. Adjust the concentration of cells as needed: add more balanced salt solution to decrease the number of red cells and white cells. The number of red cells may be increased by adding more cells from the red cell layer. Since the entire buffy coat has been utilized, it is not possible to increase the number of white cells.
11. Add 1 drop (approximately 0.05 ml) of 30 percent bovine serum albumin to each 50 ml of SSF for each 30 mg per dl total protein desired.
12. Mix well, and dispense aliquots of approximately 1.5 ml SSF into appropriate tightly stoppered containers.

---

*From Lofsness and Jensen,[24] with permission.

REFERENCES

1. Cawley, LP, et al: Immunofixation electrophoretic techniques applied to identification of proteins in serum and cerebrospinal fluid. Clin Chem 22(8):1262–1268, 1976.

2. Chow, G and Schmidley, JW: Lysis of erythrocytes and leukocytes in traumatic lumbar punctures. Arch Neurol 41:1084–1085, 1984.

3. Controni, G, et al: Cerebrospinal fluid lactic acid levels in meningitis. J Pediatr 91(3):379–384, 1977.

4. Coovadia, YM and Soliva, Z: Three latex agglutination tests compared with Gram staining for the detection of bacteria in cerebrospinal fluid. So Afr Med J 71(7):442, 1987.

5. Cutler, RWP and Spertell, RB: Cerebrospinal fluid: A selective review. Ann Neurol 11(1):1–8, 1982.

6. Davis, LE and Sperry, S: The CSF-FTA test and the significance of blood contamination. Ann Neurol 6(1):68, 1979.

7. Delmotte, P and Carton, H: Electrophoresis of cerebrospinal fluid proteins. Clin Neurol Neurosurg 83(4):183, 1981.

8. DiGiorgio, D: Determination of serum lactic dehydrogenase isoenzymes by use of the diagnostest cellulose acetate electrophoresis system. Clin Chem 17:326–331, 1971.

9. Feldman, WE: Relation of concentration of bacteria and bacterial antigen in cerebrospinal fluid to prognosis in patients with bacterial meningitis. N Engl J Med 296(8):433–435, 1977.

10. Finley, P and Wiliams, J: Assay of cerebrospinal fluid protein: A rate biuret method evaluation. Clin Chem 29(1):126–129, 1983.

11. Fishman, RA: Cerebrospinal Fluid in Diseases of the Nervous System. WB Saunders, Philadelphia, 1980.

12. Glasgow, AM and Dhiensiri, K: Improved assay for spinal fluid glutamine and values for children with Reye's syndrome. Clin Chem 20(6):642–644, 1974.

13. Glasser, L: Tapping the wealth of information in CSF. Diagnostic Medicine 4(1):23–33, 1981.

14. Glasser, L: Cells in cerebrospinal fluid. Diagnostic Medicine 4(2):33–50, 1981.

15. Godd, K: Protein estimation in spinal fluid using Coomassie blue reagent. Med Lab Sci 38:61–63, 1981.

16. Hammock, M and Milhorat, T: The cerebrospinal fluid: Current concepts of its information. Ann Clin Lab Sci 6(1):22–28, 1976.

17. Hershey, LA and Trotter, JL: The use and abuse of the cerebrospinal fluid IgG profile in the adult: A practical evaluation. Ann Neurol 8(4):426–434, 1980.

18. Hourani, BT, Hamlin, EM, and Reynolds, TB: Cerebrospinal fluid glutamine as a measure of hepatic encephalopathy. Arch Intern Med 127:1033–1036, 1971.

19. Jaffe, HW: The laboratory diagnosis of syphilis: New concepts. Ann Intern Med 83(6):846–850, 1975.

20. Johnson, KP et al: Agarose electrophoresis of cerebrospinal fluid in multiple sclerosis. Neurology 27:273–277, 1977.

21. Kjeldsberg, CP and Knight, JA: Body Fluids: Laboratory Examination of Amniotic, Cerebrospinal, Seminal, Synovial and Serous Fluids: A Textbook Atlas. American Society of Clinical Pathologists, Chicago, 1986.

22. Kjeldsberg, CP and Krieg, A: Cerebrospinal fluid and other body fluids. In Henry, JB (ed): Clinical Diagnosis and Management by Laboratory Methods. WB Saunders, Philadelphia, 1984.

23. Kolmel, HW: Atlas of Cerebrospinal Fluid Cells. Springer-Verlag, New York, 1976.

24. Lofsness, KG and Jensen, TL: The preparation of simulated spinal fluid for teaching purposes. Am J Med Technol 49(7):493–497, 1983.

25. Lopez, A et al: Suitability of solid-phase chemistry for quantification of leukocytes in cerebrospinal, seminal and peritoneal fluid. Clin Chem 33(8):1475–1476, 1987.

26. Matthews, W and Frommeyer, W: The in vitro behavior of erythrocytes in human cerebrospinal fluid. J Lab Clin Med 45:508–515, 1955.

27. McComb, JG: Recent research into the nature of cerebrospinal fluid formation and absorption. J Neurosurg 59:369–383, 1983.

28. Menkes, J: The causes of low spinal fluid sugar in bacterial meningitis: Another look. Pediatrics 44(1):1–3, 1969.

29. Murray, PR and Hampton, CM: Recovery of pathogenic bacteria from cerebrospinal fluid. J Clin Microbiol 12:554–557, 1980.

30. Nachum, R and Neely, M: Clinical diagnostic usefulness of the limulus amobocyte lysate assay. Lab Med 13(2):112–117, 1982.

31. Nagda, KK: Procoagulant activity of cerebrospinal fluid in health and disease. Indian J Med Res 74:107–110, 1981.

32. Nelson, PV, Carey, WF, and Pollard, AC: Diagnostic significance and source of lactate dehydrogenase and its isoenzymes in cerebrospinal fluid of children with a variety of neurological disorders. J Clin Pathol 28(10):828–833, 1975.

33. Novak, RW: Lack of validity of standard corrections for white blood cell counts of blood contaminated cerebrospinal fluid in infants. Am J Clin Pathol 82:95–97, 1984.

34. Osborne, J and Pizer, B: Effect on the white cell count of contaminating cerebrospinal fluid with blood. Arch Dis Child 56(5):400–401, 1981.

35. Papadopoulous, NM et al: Combined immunochemical and electrophoretic determinations of proteins in paired serum and cerebrospinal fluid samples. Clin Chem 30(11):1814–1816, 1984.

36. Plum, F and Siesjo, B: Recent advances in CSF physiology. Anesthesiology 42(6):708–729, 1975.

37. Pryce, JD, Gant, PW, and Saul, KJ: Normal concentrations of lactate, glucose and protein in cerebrospinal fluid and the diagnostic implications of abnormal concentrations. Clin Chem 16(7):562–565, 1970.

38. Reske, A, Haferkamp, G, and Hopf, H: Influence of artificial blood contamination on the analysis of cerebrospinal fluid. J Neurol 226:187–193, 1981.

39. Reunanen, MI: Spontaneous proliferation of cerebrospinal fluid mononuclear cells in multiple sclerosis. J Neuroimmunology 3:275–283, 1982.

40. Salom, I: Cryptococcal meningitis: Significance of positive antigen test on undiluted spinal fluid. NY State J Med 81(9):1369–1370, 1981.

41. Tibbling, G, Link, H, and Ohman, S: Principles of albumin and IgG analyses in neurological disorders. Scand J Lab Invest 37:385–401, 1977.

42. Tourtellotte, WW: Cerebrospinal fluid in multiple sclerosis. In Vinken, PJ and Bruyn, GW (eds): Handbook of Clinical Neurology. Elsevier, New York, 1970.

43. University of Virginia Medical Center: Clinical Laboratory Procedure Manual. Charlottesville, VA, 1988.

STUDY QUESTIONS (Choose one best answer)

1. The functions of the cerebrospinal fluid include all of the following except
   a. nutritional enrichment of nervous tissue
   b. transmittance of neurologic impulses
   c. removal of metabolic waste products
   d. protection of neurologic tissue from trauma

2. Three tubes of CSF labeled 1, 2, and 3 are received in the laboratory. They should be distributed as follows:

   a. hematology #1, chemistry #2, and microbiology #3
   b. hematology #2, chemistry #3, and microbiology #1
   c. hematology #3, chemistry #1, and microbiology #2
   d. hematology #1, chemistry #3, and microbiology #2

3. A xanthochromic CSF specimen will appear

   a. crystal clear
   b. white and turbid
   c. yellow and clear
   d. red and turbid

4. Place the appropriate letter in front of the statement that best describes CSF specimens in these two conditions.

   a. intracranial hemorrhage
   b. traumatic tap
   ____ even distribution of blood in all three tubes
   ____ xanthochromic supernatant
   ____ concentration of blood in tube 1 is greater than in tube 3
   ____ specimen contains clots

5. White blood cell counts on clear CSF specimens are performed

   a. using electronic counters
   b. only if more than 200 cells are present
   c. on undiluted specimens if there is no cell overlapping
   d. on specimens diluted 1:200 with gentian violet

6. Using a Neubauer counting chamber, 150 white blood cells are counted in 10 large squares on an undiluted CSF specimen. Calculate the WBC count.

7. To determine the WBC count on a cloudy CSF specimen that contains both red and white blood cells, it is necessary to

   a. dilute the specimen using glacial acetic acid
   b. dilute the specimen using saline
   c. determine the percentage of polynuclear and mononuclear cells in the counting chamber
   d. centrifuge the specimen prior to diluting with saline and gentian violet

8. Calculate the WBCs per microliter on a CSF specimen diluted 1:20 when 60 cells are counted in the four large squares of a Neubauer chamber.

9. White blood cell counts on CSF specimens collected during a traumatic tap

   a. should be performed using only electronic cell counters
   b. should not be performed from tubes containing streaks of blood
   c. should be corrected for white blood cells added by the traumatic tap
   d. should be corrected for both red and white blood cells added by the traumatic tap

10. Differential counts on CSF are performed on

    a. cells as they are counted in the hemocytometer
    b. coverslipped wet preparations
    c. stained smears prepared from the undiluted specimen
    d. stained smears prepared from concentrated specimens

11. In meningitis, the CSF may contain increased numbers of all of the following cells except

    a. lymphocytes
    b. ependymal
    c. monocytes
    d. neutrophils

12. Vacuolated macrophages are seen in the CSF following

    a. cerebral hemorrhage
    b. traumatic tap
    c. allergic reactions
    d. pneumoencephalography

13. Clusters of choroidal and ependymal cells are seen in the CSF in

    a. multiple sclerosis
    b. precancerous syndromes
    c. postpneumoencephalography
    d. allergic reactions

14. Chemical analysis of CSF shows that the fluid contains

    a. plasma chemicals in the same concentration as in the plasma
    b. plasma chemicals in concentrations different from those in the plasma
    c. more chemicals than are found in plasma
    d. fewer chemicals than are found in plasma

15. The normal CSF protein is

    a. 15 to 45 mg/dl
    b. 15 to 45 g/dl
    c. 50 to 100 mg/dl
    d. 50 to 100 g/dl

16. Normal CSF protein differs from serum protein by the

    a. presence of IgG
    b. presence of haptoglobin
    c. presence of ceruloplasmin
    d. absence of fibrinogen

17. Conditions that produce elevated CSF protein include all of the following except

    a. fluid leakage
    b. meningitis
    c. multiple sclerosis
    d. hemorrhage

18. Cerebrospinal fluid protein measurements obtained using a turbidity method will not represent both albumin and globulin equally if

    a. trichloroacetic acid is used
    b. sulfosalicylic acid is combined with sodium sulfate
    c. standards are made from human serum
    d. standards are made from human albumin

19. The Coomassie blue dye-binding method for measuring CSF protein is based on the principle of

    a. protein-dye precipitation
    b. protein error of indicators
    c. peptide bond and dye combination
    d. protein interference with dye binding to specific substrates

20. The IgG index is used to

    a. confirm elevated CSF protein results
    b. detect decreased levels of CSF IgG from damage to the blood-brain barrier
    c. detect increased levels of CSF IgG due to production within the central nervous system
    d. detect increased levels of serum IgG that influence the CSF concentration

21. Cerebrospinal fluid electrophoresis to confirm the diagnosis of multiple sclerosis would be expected to show

    a. increased IgG with oligoclonal bands not seen on serum electrophoresis
    b. increased IgG with oligoclonal bands similar to those seen on serum electrophoresis
    c. decreased IgG with antibody-specific oligoclonal bands
    d. decreased IgG with antibody-specific oligoclonal bands resembling those seen on serum electrophoresis

22. The normal CSF glucose is

    a. 25 to 50 mg/dl
    b. 80 to 120 mg/dl
    c. 60 to 70 percent of the blood glucose
    d. 10 to 20 percent higher than the blood glucose

23. The primary cause of decreased CSF glucose in bacterial meningitis is

    a. utilization of glucose by the microorganisms present in the fluid
    b. rapid glycolysis
    c. utilization of glucose by leukocytes present in the fluid
    d. alteration of blood-brain glucose transport

24. Measurement of CSF lactate levels is valuable for all of the following except

    a. preliminary diagnosis of tubercular meningitis
    b. preliminary diagnosis of fungal meningitis
    c. monitoring the effects of antibiotic treatment
    d. distinguishing between tubercular and fungal meningitis

25. A major CSF chemical that is measured in suspected cases of Reye's syndrome is

    a. glucose
    b. glutamine
    c. lactate
    d. lactic dehydrogenase

26. Lactic dehydrogenase isoenzymes appearing in the CSF are derived from

    a. damage to the blood-brain barrier
    b. contamination due to traumatic tap
    c. neutrophils and lymphocytes
    d. neutrophils, lymphocytes, and brain cells

27. Gram stains performed on CSF specimens are of value in the

    a. diagnosis of tubercular meningitis
    b. diagnosis of bacterial meningitis
    c. detection of viral meningitis
    d. detection of bacterial and fungal meningitis

28. Specimens from patients suspected of having fungal meningitis should be tested with

    a. Gram stain, acid-fast stain, and India ink
    b. Gram stain and India ink
    c. India ink only
    d. acid-fast stain and India ink

29. The Limulus lysate test will detect the presence of

    a. gram-positive bacteria
    b. gram-negative bacteria
    c. acid-fast organisms
    d. all microorganisms

30. The serologic test for syphilis recommended for testing CSF is the

    a. VDRL
    b. RPR
    c. FTA-ABS
    d. TPI

CASE STUDIES

1. Mary Howard, age 5, is admitted to the pediatrics ward with a temperature of 105°F, lethargy, and cervical rigidity. A lumbar spinal tap is performed, and three tubes of cloudy CSF are delivered to the laboratory. Preliminary tests results are
   WBC count: 4000 cells/μl
   Differential: 90% neutrophils, 10% lymphocytes
   Glucose: 10 mg/dl
   Protein: 150 mg/dl
   Gram stain: no organisms seen

   a. From these results, what preliminary diagnosis could the physician consider?
   b. Would any other tests be of value in the management of this patient?
   c. Is the Gram stain result of particular significance?

2. A clear CSF specimen from a 35-year-old patient experiencing mild motor difficulties has a white blood cell count of 22 mononuclear cells/μl and a total protein of 60 mg/dl.

   a. Are these results of any significance?
   b. If so, what additional tests might the physician order on this specimen?
   c. What is a possible diagnosis for this patient?

3. Examination of the CSF from a 50-year-old woman suspected of having meningitis reveals a moderately elevated white blood cell count consisting primarily of mononuclear cells. The physician must make a preliminary diagnosis of viral, tubercular, or fungal meningitis.

   a. Name the test that would provide the most valuable information in the diagnosis of each meningitis type, and explain its differential value.
   b. What other tests would be of value in the differentiation of each type?

MISCELLANEOUS BODY FLUIDS

LEARNING OBJECTIVES

Upon completion of this chapter, the reader will be able to

1. discuss the composition of seminal fluid
2. instruct a patient in the correct method for collecting a semen specimen
3. list the normal values for semen volume, viscosity, pH, sperm count, motility, and morphology
4. calculate a sperm count when provided with the number of sperm counted, the dilution, and the area of the counting chamber used
5. describe the method used to evaluate sperm motility
6. list three tests used to evaluate infertility that are not part of the routine semen analysis
7. list two methods for identifying a questionable fluid as semen
8. discuss the appearance and chemical composition of normal synovial fluid
9. list the five classifications of joint disorders, their pathologic significance, and the abnormal laboratory values associated with them
10. distinguish between a hemorrhagic arthritis and a traumatic aspiration
11. discuss the Ropes test, including methodology, grading, and significance
12. name four abnormal cells found in synovial fluid
13. discuss the principles of polarized and compensated polarized light and their significance in differentiating between monosodium urate and calcium pyrophosphate crystals
14. list four genera of bacteria frequently found in synovial fluid
15. define serous fluids
16. differentiate between transudates and exudates, including etiology, appearance, specific gravity, protein, and lactic dehydrogenase values
17. describe the appearance of normal pleural, pericardial, and peritoneal fluids
18. differentiate between a hemothorax and a hemorrhagic effusion
19. list three common chemical tests performed on pleural fluid and state their significance
20. state the purpose for performing a peritoneal lavage
21. list three common chemical tests performed on ascitic fluid and state their significance
22. discuss the physiology and composition of amniotic fluid
23. explain the principle and significance of the amniotic fluid bilirubin test
24. discuss the relationship of the lecithin-sphingomyelin ratio, shake test, phosphatidylglycerol, and amniotic fluid creatinine to fetal maturity
25. discuss the methodology of the sweat electrolyte test using pilocarpine iontophoresis and its role in the diagnosis of cystic fibrosis

This chapter includes sections on seminal, synovial, pleural, pericardial, peritoneal, and amniotic fluids, and there is a brief discussion of sweat analysis. Although blood, urine, and cerebrospinal fluid are the most common specimens received in the clinical laboratory, one must also be prepared to analyze a variety of other fluids that are formed throughout the body. These fluids are often associated with specific conditions or diseases and may require specialized tests in addition to the examinations routinely performed on all specimens. Also, unlike urine and blood, these fluids are not easily collected or always available in large amounts, so utmost care must be taken to ensure that as much information as possible is obtained from the specimen. This is best accomplished by providing laboratory personnel with a thorough understanding of these fluids, including their compositions, routine specialized test procedures, associated pathologies, and any unique precautions that must be taken. The tendency to treat body fluids in the same manner as blood specimens is a frequent source of errors, and specific procedures should be available for each fluid.[20]

SEMINAL FLUID

Of the fluids to be discussed in this chapter, seminal fluid is the specimen that is most frequently received in clinical laboratories. The two primary reasons for analysis are the evaluations of infertility cases and postvasectomy cases. Identification of a fluid as a semen can be useful in forensic medicine.

Seminal fluid is composed of four fractions that are contributed individually by the bulbourethral and urethral glands, the testis and epididymis, the prostate, and the seminal vesicles (Fig. 8–1). Each fraction differs in its composition, and the mixing of all four fractions during ejaculation is necessary for the production of a normal semen specimen. Spermatozoa are produced in the testis and mature in the epididymis. They account for only a small amount of the total semen volume, the majority of which is supplied by the seminal vesicles in the form of a viscous liquid that furnishes fructose and other nutrients to maintain the spermatozoa. The other significant contribution is made by the prostate and consists of a milky fluid that contains acid phosphatase and proteolytic enzymes that act on the fluid from the seminal vesicles, resulting in the coagulation and liquefaction of the semen.[5]

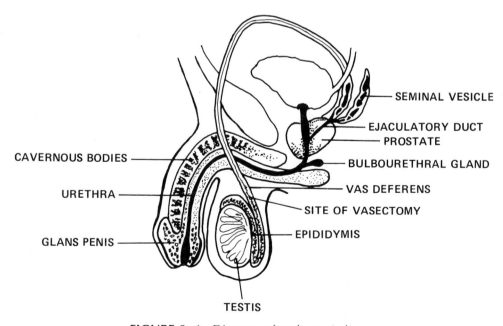

FIGURE 8–1. Diagram of male genitalia.

TABLE 8–1. Normal Values for Semen Analysis

Volume	2–5 ml
Viscosity	Pours in droplets
pH	7.3–7.8
Count	20–160 million/ml
Motility	> 50–60% within 3 hours Quality > 2.0 or fair
Morphology	< 30% Abnormal forms

The variety of the composition of the semen fractions makes proper collection of a complete specimen essential for accurate evaluation of male fertility. Patients should receive detailed instructions concerning specimen collection. Specimens should be collected in sterile containers following a 3-day period of sexual abstinence. Plastic containers are not recommended, as decreased motility has been demonstrated in specimens remaining in plastic containers for over 60 minutes.[53] The use of condoms for specimen collection is not recommended for fertility testing because the condoms may contain spermicidal agents. Postvasectomy specimens, in which only the presence of sperm—viable or nonviable—is significant, are not affected by condoms. Whenever possible, the specimen should be collected in a room provided by the laboratory. However, if this is not appropriate, the specimen should be kept at room temperature and delivered to the laboratory within 1 hour. The time of specimen collection, not specimen receipt, must be recorded by the laboratory. A fresh semen specimen is clotted and should liquefy within 30 minutes after collection; therefore, the time of collection is essential for evaluation of semen liquefaction. Analysis of the specimen cannot begin until after liquefaction has occurred. Specimens awaiting motility analysis should be kept at 37°C.

When evaluating semen specimens in cases of infertility, the following parameters are routinely measured: volume, viscosity, pH, sperm count, motility, and morphology. Normal values are shown in Table 8–1.

VOLUME AND VISCOSITY

Normal semen volume ranges between 2 and 5 ml and is measured by pouring the specimen into a graduated cylinder. Viscosity can be determined as the specimen is being poured into the cylinder. A specimen of normal viscosity will pour in droplets and will not appear clumped or stringy. Ratings of 0 (watery) to 4 (gel-like) can be assigned to the viscosity report.[37] Always be sure that the specimen has completely liquefied prior to determining viscosity. Increased viscosity or incomplete liquefaction will interfere with sperm motility. Any abnormal appearance of the fluid—such as the presence of blood, pigmentation, or increased turbidity—that may be due to white blood cells should also be noted at this time. The leukocyte esterase reagent strip test may be used to detect the presence of white blood cells.[34]

pH

The pH of normal semen is slightly alkaline, with a range of 7.3 to 7.8, and can be measured using pH-testing paper.[28] An abnormally high ratio of prostatic fluid to seminal fluid will produce a more acidic pH.[28]

Sperm Count

Even though fertilization is accomplished by one spermatozoa, the actual number of sperm present in a semen specimen is a valid measurement of fertility. Normal values are commonly listed as 20 to 160 million sperm per milliliter, with counts between 10 and 20 million per milliliter considered borderline. The sperm count is performed in the same manner as blood and CSF counts; that is, by diluting the specimen and counting the cells in a Neubauer chamber. The amount of the dilution and the number of squares counted vary among laboratories. Two frequently used methods dilute the specimen 1:20 using the method described in chapter 7 and count the sperm in either the five RBC squares or in two large WBC squares (Fig. 8–2). When the five RBC squares are used, the number of sperm counted is multiplied by 1,000,000 to calculate the number of sperm per milliliter.[28, 47] If the two WBC squares are used, the count is multiplied by 100,000 to achieve the same result.[5]

The basic cell counting formula discussed in chapter 7 can also be applied to sperm counts. But because this formula provides the number of cells per microliter, the figure must then be multiplied by 1000 to give the number of sperm per milliliter.

Example:

1. Using a 1:20 dilution, 600 sperm are counted in the two WBC counting squares. Calculate the sperm count per milliliter.

   A. 600 sperm counted $\times$ 100,000 = 60,000,000 sperm/ml

   B. $\dfrac{600 \text{ sperm} \times 20 \text{ (dilution)}}{2 \text{ (squares counted)} \times 0.1 \text{ }\mu\text{l (volume counted)}} = 60,000 \text{ sperm}/\mu\text{l}$

   60,000 sperm/μl $\times$ 1,000 = 60,000,000 sperm/ml

2. Using a 1:20 dilution, 60 sperm are counted in the five RBC counting squares. Calculate the sperm count per milliliter.

   A. 60 sperm counted $\times$ 1,000,000 = 60,000,000 sperm/ml

   B. $\dfrac{60 \text{ sperm} \times 20 \text{ (dilution)}}{5 \text{ (squares counted)} \times 0.004 \text{ }\mu\text{l (volume counted)}} = 60,000 \text{ sperm}/\mu\text{l}$

   60,000 sperm/μl $\times$ 1,000 = 60,000,000 sperm/ml

Dilution of the semen prior to counting is essential to provide for immobilization of the sperm. The traditional diluting fluid contains sodium bicarbonate and formalin, which immobilize and preserve the cells; however, good results can also be achieved using tap water.[28] Care should be taken not to contaminate the specimen with diluting fluid prior to determining the motility. Both dilutions and counts should be performed in duplicate on completely liquefied specimens to ensure accuracy.

Motility

Equal to—if not more important than—the number of sperm present is the motility of the sperm, because once presented to the cervix, the sperm must propel themselves through the fallopian tubes to the ovum. Laboratory evaluation of sperm motility is a subjective procedure that is performed by examining the undiluted specimen microscopically and determining the percentage of sperm showing active motility. Sperm should be evaluated on their progressive forward movement, and any motility owing to brownian

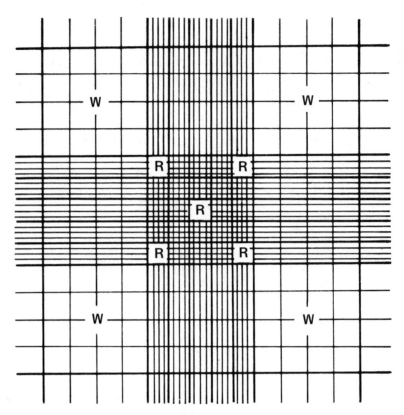

FIGURE 8–2. Areas of Neubauer counting chamber used for red and white cell counts.

movement should be disregarded. Many laboratories not only report the percentage of motile sperm but also grade the motility either on a scale of 0 to 4, with 4 indicating rapid progressive movement, or by word descriptions ranging from poor to excellent. Approximately 25 high-power fields should be examined. The percentage and quality of motility should be determined in each field, and an average of these results should be reported. Various time frames have been established for the determination of motility, with some laboratories testing the specimen at periodic intervals up to 24 hours. However, the common practice is to observe motility within 3 hours of collection but not before liquefaction has taken place. A minimum motility of 50 to 60 percent with a quality of fair (2.0) is considered normal for specimens tested within the 3-hour time period.

MORPHOLOGY

Just as the presence of a normal number of sperm that are nonmotile will produce infertility, the presence of sperm that are morphologically incapable of fertilization also will result in infertility. Sperm morphology is evaluated with respect to both head and tail appearance. The normal sperm has an oval head measuring approximately 3 × 5 μm and a long, tapering tail **(Color Plate 73)**. Abnormalities in head structure (Fig. 8–3) are associated with poor ovum penetration and include double heads, giant and amorphous heads, pinheads, tapering heads, and constricted heads. Motility is impeded in sperm with double or coiled tails. Immature sperm (spermatids) also may be present and must be differentiated from white blood cells. They are more spherical than mature sperm and may or may not have tails. The presence of a high number of immature forms is considered abnormal because sperm usually mature within the epididymis prior to their release. Sperm morphology should be reported from a stained specimen examined under oil immersion. The recommended stain is the Papanicolaou. However, if this is not available, acceptable results can be obtained by using hematoxylin, crystal violet, or Giemsa

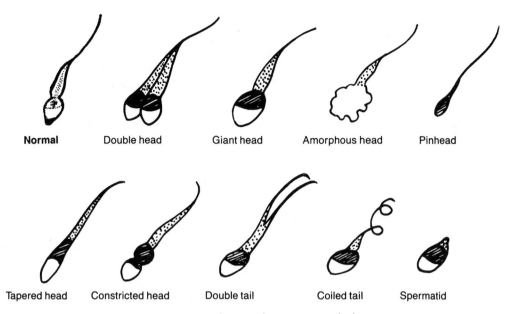

Normal Double head Giant head Amorphous head Pinhead

Tapered head Constricted head Double tail Coiled tail Spermatid

FIGURE 8–3. Abnormal sperm morphology.

stains.[13] At least 200 spermatozoa should be examined, and the percentage of abnormal forms should be reported. A specimen that contains less than 30 percent abnormal forms is considered normal.

Should abnormalities be discovered in any of these routine parameters, additional tests may be requested (Table 8–2). The most common are tests for sperm viability, seminal fluid fructose level, and sperm agglutinins. Concern about the viability of sperm arises when a specimen has a normal count and markedly decreased motility. Viability is tested by mixing the specimen with an eosin-nigrosin stain and examining microscopically for dead cells that stain red against a purple background. Living cells are not infiltrated by the eosin dye and remain a bluish-white color. Low sperm counts may be caused by a lack of support medium produced in the seminal vesicles, which is indicated by a low to absent fructose level in the semen specimen. Sperm agglutinating antibodies may be present in the plasma of either the male or his female partner and will result in the clumping and inactivation of the sperm. The presence of antibodies in the male plasma can be suspected when clumps of sperm are observed during a routine semen analysis; whereas the presence of antisperm antibodies in the female partner will result in a normal semen analysis accompanied by continued infertility. Confirmation of sperm agglutinating antibodies is accomplished by mixing the semen specimen with the appropriate male or female serum and observing the agglutination or immobilization of the sperm.[13] Quantitation of antispermatozoa antibodies can be performed with solid-phase radioimmunoassay using ^{125}I bacterial protein-A.[8]

Postvasectomy semen analysis is a much less involved procedure when compared with the infertility analysis, inasmuch as the only concern is the presence or absence of spermatozoa. The length of time required for complete sterilization to occur can vary greatly among patients and depends on both time and number of ejaculations. Therefore, it is not uncommon to find viable sperm in a postvasectomy patient, and care should be taken not to overlook even a single sperm. Specimens are routinely tested at monthly intervals beginning at 2 months postvasectomy and continuing until 2 consecutive monthly specimens show no spermatozoa. Recommended testing includes microscopic examination of samples from both the mixed undiluted specimen and sediment from the centrifuged specimen.[47]

On certain occasions, the laboratory may be called upon to determine whether semen is actually present in a specimen. A primary example of this is in cases of alleged

TABLE 8–2. Additional Testing for Abnormal Semen Analysis

ABNORMAL RESULT	POSSIBLE ABNORMALITY	TEST
Decreased motility with normal count	Viability	Eosin-nigrosin stain
Decreased count	Lack of seminal vesicle support medium	Fructose level
Decreased motility with clumping	Male antisperm antibodies	Sperm agglutination with male plasma
Normal analysis with continued infertility	Female antisperm antibodies	Sperm agglutination with female plasma

rape. It may be possible to microscopically examine the specimen for the presence of sperm, with best results being obtained by enhancing the specimen with xylene and examining under phase microscopy.[12] However, a more reliable procedure is to test the material chemically for acid phosphatase content. Because seminal fluid is the only body fluid with a high concentration of acid phosphatase, the detection of this enzyme can confirm the presence of semen in a specimen. Further information can often be obtained by performing ABO blood grouping, HLA testing, and DNA analysis on the specimen.

SYNOVIAL FLUID

Synovial fluid, often referred to as "joint fluid," is a viscous liquid found in the joint cavities (Fig. 8–4). It is formed as an ultrafiltrate of the plasma across the synovial membrane, into which a mucopolysaccharide containing hyaluronic acid and a small amount of protein is secreted by the cells of the synovial membrane. Except for high-molecular-weight proteins, the plasma filtration is nonselective; therefore, normal synovial fluid has essentially the same chemical composition as the plasma. Synovial fluid supplies nutrients to the cartilage and acts as a lubricant to the surfaces of the frequently moving joints.

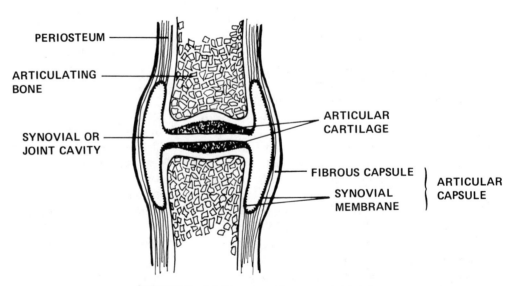

FIGURE 8–4. Diagram of a synovial joint.

COLLECTION

Although the fluid is found in all joints, the specimen usually received in the laboratory is an aspirate of the knee. Synovial fluid is collected by needle aspiration, called arthrocentesis. The normal amount of fluid contained in the knee cavity is less than 3.5 ml; however, this amount increases in disorders of the joints.[14] Therefore, the volume of fluid collected is dependent on the degree of fluid buildup in the joints. Normal synovial fluid will not clot; however, fluid from a diseased joint may contain fibrinogen and form a clot. Both anticoagulated and nonanticoagulated specimens should be collected. Recommended specimen containers include those enumerated below.[42]

1. Ethylenediaminetetraacetic acid (EDTA) (sequestrin) tube for cell counts and differentials. When using commercially prepared EDTA tubes, the specified amount of fluid should be added because artifacts may occur if too little fluid is mixed with the anticoagulant.
2. Heparinized tube for chemical and immunologic tests. Specimens should be centrifuged and the fluid separated from the cells as soon as possible to prevent the addition of intracellular constituents to the fluid. Fluid for complement studies should be frozen before storage.
3. Plain, sterile tube for microbiologic testing and crystal examination.

Analysis of synovial fluid is used to classify joint disorders in terms of their pathologic origins.[43] The five commonly used categories associated with fluid buildup and arthritis and their clinical significance are listed in Table 8–3. Results from both synovial fluid and blood analyses must be considered along with the patient's clinical history before a category is assigned (Table 8–4).

SYNOVIAL FLUID IN THE HEMATOLOGY LABORATORY

The major portion of the routine synovial fluid analysis takes place in the hematology laboratory and includes a report of the appearance, viscosity, cell count, cell differential, and crystal identification. Normal synovial fluid appears clear and pale yellow. The color becomes a deeper yellow in the presence of inflammation and may have a greenish tinge with bacterial infection. As with CSF, the presence of blood from a hemorrhagic arthritis must be distinguished from blood from a traumatic aspiration. This is accomplished primarily by observing the uneven distribution of blood in the specimens obtained from a traumatic aspiration. Turbidity occurs when the cell count is elevated and is usually proportional to the number of cells present. However, a milky fluid may also indicate the presence of crystals. A report of the gross appearance is an essential part of the laboratory report.[20]

TABLE 8–3. Classification and Pathologic Significance of Joint Disorders[43]

GROUP CLASSIFICATION	PATHOLOGIC SIGNIFICANCE
I. Noninflammatory	Degenerative joint disorders
II. Inflammatory	Immunologic problems, including rheumatoid arthritis and lupus erythematosus
III. Septic	Microbial infection
IV. Crystal-induced	Gout Pseudogout
V. Hemorrhagic	Traumatic injury Coagulation deficiencies

TABLE 8–4. Summary of Laboratory Findings in Joint Disorders[14, 30, 43]

GROUP CLASSIFICATION	LABORATORY FINDINGS
I. Noninflammatory	Clear, yellow fluid Good viscosity WBCs less than 5000 Neutrophils less than 30% Normal glucose (similar to blood glucose)
II. Inflammatory	Cloudy, yellow fluid Poor viscosity WBCs 2,000 to 100,000 Neutrophils greater than 50% Decreased glucose Possible auto-antibodies present
III. Septic	Cloudy, yellow-green fluid Poor viscosity WBCs 10,000 to 200,000 Neutrophils greater than 90% Decreased glucose Positive culture
IV. Crystal-induced	Cloudy or milky fluid Poor viscosity WBCs 500 to 200,000 Neutrophils less than 90% Decreased glucose Elevated uric acid Crystals present
V. Hemorrhagic	Cloudy, red fluid Poor viscosity WBCs less than 5000 Neutrophils less than 50% Normal glucose RBCs present

Viscosity of the synovial fluid comes from the polymerization of the hyaluronic acid and is essential for the proper lubrication of the joints. Arthritis affects both the production of hyaluronate and its ability to polymerize, thus decreasing the viscosity of the fluid. Several methods are used to measure the viscosity of the fluid, the simplest being to observe the ability of the fluid to form a string from the tip of a syringe. A string that measures 4 to 6 cm is considered normal. The laboratory may be requested to measure the degree of hyaluronate polymerization by performing a Ropes, or mucin clot, test. When added to a solution of 2 to 5 percent acetic acid, normal synovial fluid will form a solid clot surrounded by clear fluid. As the ability of the hyaluronate to polymerize decreases, the clot becomes less firm and the surrounding fluid increases in turbidity. The Ropes test is reported in terms of good (solid clot), fair (soft clot), poor (friable clot), and very poor (no clot).[54]

Both red and white blood cell counts should be performed on all specimens unless the presence of red blood cells is known to be due to a traumatic tap. Manual counts on thoroughly mixed specimens are done using the Neubauer counting chamber in the same manner as CSF and sperm counts. Clear fluids can usually be counted undiluted, but dilutions are necessary when fluids are turbid or bloody. Dilutions can be made using the procedure presented in chapter 7; however, traditional WBC diluting fluid cannot be used because it contains acetic acid, which will cause the formation of mucin clots. Normal saline can be used as a diluent. If it is necessary to lyse the red blood cells, hypotonic saline or saline that contains saponin is a suitable diluent. Methylene blue added to the normal saline will stain the white cell nuclei, permitting separation of the red and white cells during counts performed on mixed specimens. The use of phase rather than light microscopy also will aid in distinguishing between the two cell types.[42] Electronic cell counters should not be used for synovial fluid cell counts because the viscous fluid may clot the tubing and the presence of tissue cells can falsely elevate counts. The normal synovial fluid red blood cell count is 0 to 2000 cells per microliter. White blood cell counts below 200 cells per microliter are considered normal and may reach 100,000 cells per microliter or higher in severe inflammations.[35]

Mononuclear cells, including lymphocytes, monocytes, macrophages, and synovial tissue cells, are the primary cells seen in normal synovial fluid. Neutrophils should account for less than 25 percent of the differential count. Increased neutrophils indicate a septic condition; whereas an elevated cell count with a predominance of lymphocytes suggests a nonseptic inflammation. In both normal and abnormal specimens, cells may appear more vacuolated than they do on a blood smear.[29] Besides increased numbers of these usually normal cells, other cell abnormalities include the presence of LE cells; Reiter cells (vacuolated macrophages with ingested neutrophils); and RA cells, or ragocytes (neutrophils with small, dark, cytoplasmic granules that consist of precipitated rheumatoid factor).[3, 39] Differential counts should be performed on thinly smeared Wright-stained slides; however, an estimate of the percentage of neutrophils present can be obtained from the counting chamber when the diluting fluid contains methylene blue.[29] Table 8–5 summarizes the most frequently encountered cells and inclusions seen in synovial fluid.

Microscopic examination of synovial fluid for the presence of crystals is used in the diagnosis of crystal-induced arthritis. The primary crystals seen in synovial fluid are monosodium urate (uric acid), which is found in cases of gout, and calcium pyrophosphate, which is associated with cases of pseudogout. Cholesterol crystals, crystals of apatite (the major mineral found in cartilage), and corticosteroid crystals resulting from drug injections also may be seen. The microscopic characteristics of these crystals are listed in Table 8–6. It is recommended that crystal examination be performed soon after the fluid is collected, because changes in temperature and pH in the fluid can affect crystal solubility, producing erroneous results. Refrigeration of specimens decreases the solubility of uric acid, resulting in an increase in monosodium urate crystals. Likewise, a rise in pH due to the loss of carbon dioxide upon exposure to room air encourages the formation of calcium phosphate crystals.[9]

Fluid should be examined unstained, under both direct and compensated polarized light for better visualization and identification of monosodium urate and calcium pyrophosphate crystals. Monosodium urate crystals are seen routinely as needle-shaped crystals, often found within the cytoplasm of neutrophils **(Color Plate 74)**. Calcium pyrophosphate crystals may appear rhombic-shaped **(Color Plate 75)** but can also be found as intracellular needles. By examining the refractive properties of the crystals under compensated polarized light, it is possible to differentiate between the two needle-shaped crystals. The basic principle of polarized light is illustrated in Figure 8–5. As can be seen from the diagram, the crystal must be able to bend the light waves (B) that pass through the analyzer. When this happens, the crystal will appear white against a black background. Both monosodium urate and calcium pyrophosphate crystals will polarize direct light; however, monosodium urate will appear brighter against the black background due to its strong birefringence (ability to break the light beam into two rays).

Once the presence of crystals has been determined using direct polarized light, positive identification can be made by examining the slide under compensated polarized light. A first-order red compensator is placed in the microscope between the crystal and

TABLE 8–5. Cells and Inclusions Seen in Synovial Fluid

CELL/INCLUSION	DESCRIPTION	SIGNIFICANCE
Neutrophil	Polymorphonuclear leukocyte	Bacterial sepsis Crystal-induced inflammation
Lymphocyte	Mononuclear leukocyte	Nonseptic inflammation
Macrophage (monocyte)	Large mononuclear leukocyte, may be vacuolated	Normal Viral infections
Synovial lining cell	Similar to macrophage, but may be multinucleated, resembling a mesothelial cell	Normal
LE cell	Neutrophil containing characteristic ingested "round body"	Lupus erythematosus
Reiter cell	Vacuolated macrophage with ingested neutrophils	Reiter's syndrome Nonspecific inflammation
RA cell (ragocyte)	Neutrophil with dark cytoplasmic granules containing immune complexes	Rheumatoid arthritis Immunologic inflammation
Cartilage cells	Large, multinucleated cells	Osteoarthritis
Rice bodies	Macroscopically resemble polished rice Microscopically show collagen and fibrin	Tuberculosis, septic and rheumatoid arthritis
Fat droplets	Refractile intracellular and extracellular globules Stain with Sudan dyes	Traumatic injury
Hemosiderin	Inclusions with synovial cells	Pigmented villonodular synovitis

the analyzer (see Fig. 8–5). The red compensator separates the light beam into slow- and fast-moving components and retards red light so that the background becomes red instead of black. Monosodium urate and calcium pyrophosphate crystals exhibit different birefringent properties when light has been separated into slow and fast vibrations, and identification can be made by observing the colors that the crystals produce. When monosodium urate is aligned with the slow vibration, it appears yellow, a sign of negative birefringence; whereas calcium pyrophosphate is blue and positively birefringent (**Color Plates 76 and 77**). Likewise, when the crystals are aligned opposite the slow vibration, monosodium urate will appear blue and calcium pyrophosphate will appear yellow (Fig. 8–6). Care must be taken to align the crystals in accordance with the direction of slow vibration shown on the compensator. Patterns that vary from those shown in Figure 8–6 may indicate the presence of one of the less common crystals, and additional testing and the patient's history must be considered.

TABLE 8–6. Synovial Fluid Crystals*

CRYSTAL	SHAPE		COMPENSATED POLARIZED LIGHT	LOCATION
Monosodium urate	Needles		Negative birefringence	Intracellular and extracellular
Calcium pyrophosphate	Rods Needles Rhombics		Positive birefringence	Intracellular and extracellular
Cholesterol	Notched rhombic plates		Negative birefringence	Extracellular
Apatite	Small needles		May need electron microscope	Intracellular and extracellular
Corticosteroid	Flat, variable shaped plates		Positive and negative birefringence	Primarily intracellular

*Adapted from Samuelson and Ward.[48]

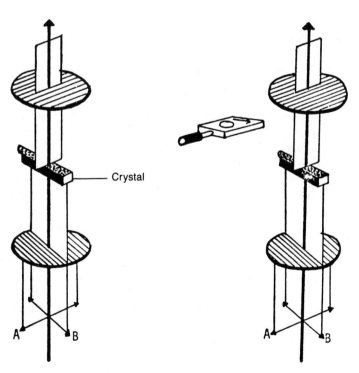

FIGURE 8–5. *(Left)* Direct polarized light. *(Right)* Compensated polarized light. (Adapted from Phelps, Steele, and McCarty.[40])

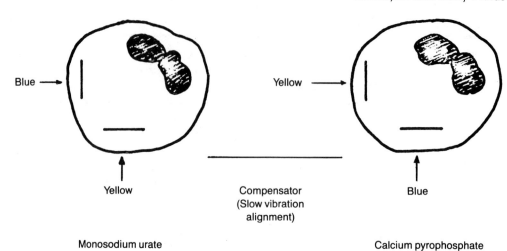

FIGURE 8–6. Crystals under compensated polarized light.

SYNOVIAL FLUID IN THE CHEMISTRY LABORATORY

Because synovial fluid is chemically an ultrafiltrate of plasma, chemistry test values are approximately the same as serum values. Therefore, few chemistry tests are considered clinically important. The most frequently requested test is the glucose determination, because markedly decreased values are indicative of inflammatory (group II) or septic (group III) disorders. Because normal synovial fluid glucose values are based on the blood glucose level, simultaneous blood and synovial fluid samples should be obtained, preferably after the patient has fasted for 8 hours to allow equilibration between the two fluids. Under these conditions, normal synovial fluid glucose should not be more than 10 mg per dl lower than the blood value.[14]

Recently, measurement of synovial fluid lactate levels has been shown to provide rapid differentiation between inflammatory and septic arthritis and does not require equilibration and comparison with blood lactate levels. Synovial fluid lactate levels below 7.5 mmole per liter provide a 98 percent exclusion for septic arthritis; whereas levels above 7.5 mmole per liter are found consistently with septic arthritis but may also be seen in rheumatoid arthritis.[7]

Other chemistry tests that may be requested are the total protein and uric acid determinations. Because the large protein molecules are not filtered through the synovial membranes, normal synovial fluid contains less than 3 g per dl of protein (approximately one third of the serum value). Increased levels are found in inflammatory and hemorrhagic disorders; however, measurement of synovial fluid protein does not contribute greatly to the classification of these disorders.[30] When requested, the analysis is performed using the same methods used for serum protein determinations. The elevation of serum uric acid in cases of gout is well known; therefore, demonstration of an elevated synovial fluid uric acid may be used to confirm the diagnosis when the presence of crystals cannot be demonstrated in the fluid.

In some laboratories, the performance of the Ropes viscosity test, discussed in the hematology section above, is the responsibility of the chemistry department, as is the observation of spontaneous clotting when unheparinized specimens are received.

SYNOVIAL FLUID IN THE MICROBIOLOGY LABORATORY

Although the primary role of the microbiology laboratory is to identify the organisms causing septic inflammations, Gram stains and cultures should be performed on all synovial fluid specimens because infection may occur as a secondary complication of any inflammation.[29] Bacterial infections are most frequently seen; however, fungal, tubercular, and viral infections also can occur. When they are suspected, special culturing procedures should be utilized. Routine bacterial cultures should always include an enrichment medium, such as chocolate agar, because in addition to *Staphylococcus* and *Streptococcus*, the most common genera that infect synovial fluid are the fastidious *Hemophilus* and *Neisseria*.

SYNOVIAL FLUID IN THE SEROLOGY LABORATORY

Due to the association of the immune system to the inflammation process, the serology laboratory plays an important role in the diagnosis of joint disorders. However, the majority of the tests are performed on serum, with actual analysis of the synovial fluid serving as a confirmatory measure in cases that are difficult to diagnose. The autoimmune diseases rheumatoid arthritis and lupus erythematosus cause very serious inflammation of the joints and are diagnosed in the serology laboratory by demonstrating the presence of their particular autoantibodies in the patient's serum. These same antibodies can also be demonstrated in the synovial fluid, if necessary.

Determination of synovial fluid complement levels can be an aid in the differential diagnosis of arthritis as to immunologic and nonimmunologic origin. Measurement of the complement components C1q, C4, C2, and C3 is performed primarily by single radial immunodiffusion.[36] Under normal and nonimmunologic conditions, synovial fluid complement levels parallel the fluid protein levels. Therefore, to ensure that abnormal complement levels are not due to changes in synovial membrane filtration, complement values must be expressed as their ratio to synovial fluid protein.[4]

SEROUS FLUIDS

The closed cavities of the body—namely, the pleural, pericardial, and peritoneal cavities—are each lined by two membranes referred to as the serous membranes. One membrane lines the cavity wall (parietal membrane), and the other covers the organs within the cavity (visceral membrane). The fluid between the membranes, which provides lubrication as the surfaces move against each other, is called serous fluid. Normally only a small amount of serous fluid is present because production and reabsorption take place at a constant rate.

FORMATION

Serous fluids are formed as ultrafiltrates of plasma, with no additional material contributed by the membrane cells. The small amount of filtered protein is removed by the lymphatic system. Production and reabsorption are subject to hydrostatic and colloidal (oncotic) pressures from the capillaries serving the cavities. Under normal conditions, colloidal pressure from serum proteins is the same in the capillaries on both sides of the membrane. Therefore, the greater hydrostatic pressure in the systemic capillaries on the parietal side favors fluid production through the parietal membrane and reabsorption through the visceral membrane. Figure 8–7 demonstrates the normal formation and absorption of pleural fluid.

Fluids for laboratory examination are collected by needle aspiration from the respective cavities. These aspiration procedures are referred to as thoracentesis (pleural), pericardiocentesis (pericardial), and paracentesis (peritoneal). Abundant fluid is usually collected; therefore, suitable specimens are available for each section of the laboratory. An anticoagulated specimen is needed for cell counts, a sterile tube for culture, and a nonanticoagulated specimen for observation of spontaneous clotting. Large volumes of fluid should be concentrated prior to microbiologic and cytologic examinations.

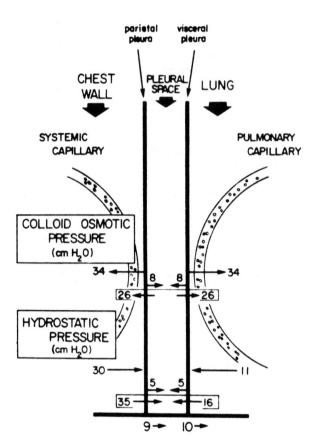

FIGURE 8–7. The normal formation and absorption of pleural fluid. (From Fraser and Pare,[11] p 2069, with permission.)

TRANSUDATES AND EXUDATES

Many pathologic conditions can cause a buildup (effusion) of serous fluid. However, a general classification of the cause of the effusion can be accomplished by separating the fluid into the category of transudate or exudate. Effusions that form because of a systemic disorder that disrupts the balance in the regulation of fluid filtration and reabsorption—such as the changes in hydrostatic pressure created by congestive heart failure—are called transudates. Exudates are produced by conditions that directly involve the membranes of the particular cavity, including infections and malignancies. Transudates also can be thought of as resulting from a mechanical process, and exudates from an inflammatory process. Classification of a serous fluid as to transudate or exudate can provide a valuable initial step in the diagnosis and in the course of laboratory testing, as further testing of transudate fluids is usually not necessary.[25]

A variety of laboratory tests have been used to differentiate between transudates and exudates, including appearance, specific gravity, total protein, lactic dehydrogenase, cell counts, and spontaneous clotting. Differential values for these parameters are shown in Table 8–7.

As can be seen using these criteria, one would expect a transudate to be a clear fluid with a specific gravity less than 1.015, protein less than 3.0 g per dl, and a lactic dehydrogenase below 200 IU.

Traditionally, specific gravity and protein were considered to be the most valuable criteria for classification. But in recent years, the lactic dehydrogenase has replaced the specific gravity.[32] Fluid-to-blood ratios for protein and lactic dehydrogenase have provided greater reliability in the differentiation.[24] As shown in Table 8–8, a combination of the fluid to blood protein ratio, lactic dehydrogenase, and fluid to blood lactic dehydrogenase ratio can provide 100 percent fluid-to-blood reliability.

TABLE 8–7. Laboratory Differentiation of Transudates and Exudates

	TRANSUDATE	EXUDATE
Appearance	Clear	Cloudy
Specific gravity	< 1.015	> 1.015
Total protein	< 3.0 g/dl	> 3.0 g/dl
Fluid: serum protein ratio	< 0.5	> 0.5
Lactic dehydrogenase	< 200 IU	> 200 IU
Fluid: serum LD ratio	< 0.6	> 0.6
Cell count	< 1000/µl	> 1000/µl
Spontaneous clotting	No	Possible

TABLE 8–8. Classification of Exudates and Transudates*

CRITERIA	EXUDATE		TRANSUDATE	
	CORRECT	MISDIAGNOSED	CORRECT	MISDIAGNOSED
Specific gravity 1.016	55 (87.3%)	8 (12.7%)	29 (78.3%)	8 (21.7%)
Pleural fluid protein 3G%	57 (90.4%)	6 (9.6%)	32 (86.4%)	5 (13.6%)
Pleural fluid protein and blood protein ratio 0.5	59 (93.6%)	4 (6.4%)	36 (97.3%)	1 (2.7%)
Pleural fluid LDH and blood LDH ratio 0.6	56 (88.8%)	7 (11.2%)	35 (94.6%)	2 (5.4%)
Pleural fluid LDH 200 I.U.	45 (73.0%)	18 (27.0%)	36 (97.3%)	1 (2.7%)
Pleural fluid glucose 90 mgm%	42 (66.6%)	21 (33.4%)	35 (94.6%)	2 (5.4%)
Pleural fluid WBC-1000	48 (77.9%)	15 (22.1%)	30 (81.0%)	7 (19.0%)
Protein ratio/LDH	61 (96.8%)	2 (3.2%)	37 (100.0%)	0
Protein ratio/LDH ratio	59 (93.6%)	4 (6.4%)	36 (97.3%)	1 (2.7%)
Protein ratio/LDH/ LDH ratio	63 (100.0%)	0	37 (100.0%)	0

*From Jain, Gupta, and Kahn,[24] p 824, with permission.

General Laboratory Procedures

Routine fluid examination—including classification as a transudate or exudate, appearance, cell count and differential, and chemistry and microbiology procedures—is performed in the same manner on all serous fluids. However, the significance of the test results and the need for specialized tests vary among fluids; therefore, the interpretation of routine and special procedures will be discussed individually for each of the three serous fluids.

Cell counts are usually performed manually using the Neubauer counting chamber and the methods discussed in chapter 7. When performing white cell counts on grossly bloody specimens with high protein levels, the red cells should be lysed using hypotonic saline or saline with saponin. This will prevent any unusual clumping or clotting of the fluid. Some laboratories use electronic cell counters for high counts, but corrections must be made for the inclusion of tissue cells in the count, and care must be taken to prevent the blocking of tubing with fluid debris. Differential counts are performed on Wright-stained smears. Any suspicious cells seen on the differential should be referred to the cytology laboratory or the pathologist.

Pleural Fluid

Formation

Abnormal accumulation of pleural fluid (or any serous fluid) will occur when conditions that affect capillary hydrostatic pressure, colloidal pressure, permeability, and lymphatic drainage are present. Examples in each of these cases include congestive heart failure, hypoalbuminemia, pneumonia, and carcinoma.[46] Congestive heart failure and hypoalbuminemia are systemic disorders that result in production of transudate fluid; whereas pneumonia and carcinoma cause localized damage with exudative effusions. Therefore, differentiation of the fluid into the category of transudate or exudate can be significant.

Appearance

Considerable diagnostic information concerning the etiology of a pleural effusion can be learned from the appearance of the specimen. Normal and transudate pleural fluids are clear and pale yellow. Turbidity is usually related to the presence of white blood cells and indicates bacterial infection, tuberculosis, or an immunologic disorder, such as rheumatoid arthritis. The presence of blood in the pleural fluid can signify a hemothorax (traumatic injury), membrane damage such as occurs in malignancy, or may be due to a traumatic aspiration. As seen with other fluids, blood from a traumatic tap appears streaked and uneven. To differentiate between a hemothorax and hemorrhagic exudate, it is necessary to run a hematocrit on the fluid. If the blood is from a hemothorax, the fluid hematocrit will be similar to the whole blood hematocrit because the effusion is actually occurring from the inpouring of blood from the injury. A chronic membrane disease effusion will contain both blood and increased pleural fluid, resulting in a much lower hematocrit.[29] The appearance of a milky pleural fluid may be due to the presence of chylous material from thoracic duct leakage or to pseudochylous material produced in chronic inflammatory conditions. To distinguish between the two substances, the fluid is mixed with ether. True chylous material will be extracted into the ether, leaving a clear layer of fluid.[30] Also, Sudan III staining will be positive with chylous material and negative with pseudochylous material.

White blood cell and differential counts are routinely performed on pleural fluids and are useful in the diagnosis of tuberculosis and bacterial infections. Counts above 1000 cells per μl are considered elevated.[29] Tubercular effusions show moderately elevated counts with a predominance of lymphocytes and the presence of plasma cells (**Color Plate 78**). In bacterial infections, the count is usually higher, and neutrophils are the predominant cell. Increased lymphocytes are also frequently seen in malignant effusions.[33] Although cytologic examination is usually requested separately, the differential smear should be examined for the presence of both normal and abnormal cells. Besides the normal and abnormal cells seen on blood differentials, pleural fluid specimens may also contain macrophages, histiocytes, mesothelial cells, and malignant tissue cells. Mesothelial cells from the pleural membranes can appear in a variety of forms **(Color Plates 79 and 80)**. They are increased in nonseptic inflammations but are seldom seen in tuberculosis and bacterial infections. Care must be taken not to confuse mesothelial cells with malignant cells, and any questionable cells should be referred to the pathologist **(Color Plates 81 to 84)**.

Because pleural fluid is strictly a plasma ultrafiltrate, normal chemistry values are the same as the plasma levels. Besides the chemical tests used to differentiate transudates and exudates, the most common chemical tests performed on pleural fluid are glucose, pH, and amylase. Decreased glucose levels are seen in tubercular and rheumatoid inflammations.[21] The demonstration of a low fluid pH is of some value in the diagnosis of pneumonia, tuberculosis, and malignancy and may indicate the need for chest drainage. The finding of a pH as low as 6.0 indicates an esophageal rupture.[23] As with serum, elevated amylase levels are associated with pancreatic disorders, and amylase is often first elevated in the pleural fluid. Therefore, amylase determinations are recommended procedures on all pleural fluids of questionable etiology. Table 8–9 summarizes the laboratory results for some of the more frequently encountered pleural effusions.

Serologic testing of pleural fluid is used to differentiate effusions of immunologic and malignant origin from those of noninflammatory and nonmalignant origin. The testing includes antinuclear antibody tests, quantitation of immunoglobulins, complement components, and carcinoembryonic antigen (CEA). Increased levels of immunoglobulins and CEA or decreased complement is indicative of inflammatory and neoplastic reactions. Increased CEA levels provide the best diagnostic information because they are closely associated with malignancy.[1]

PERICARDIAL FLUID

Normally, only a small amount (10 to 50 ml) of clear, pale-yellow fluid is found between the pericardial membranes.[30] Pericardial effusions are primarily the result of changes in the permeability of the membranes due to infection (pericarditis), malignancy, or metabolic damage. The presence of an effusion is suspected when cardiac compression is noted during the physician's examination.

Aspirated fluid will appear clear in metabolic disorders. However, turbid fluids, which are produced by infection and malignancy, are more commonly encountered. Milky fluid is seen when damage to the lymphatic system has occurred. Blood-streaked fluid is frequently present when membrane damage is caused by tuberculosis and tumors. Grossly bloody effusions are seen in cardiac puncture and misuse of anticoagulant drugs.

White blood cell counts over 1000 cells per μl are indicative of infection. As with pleural fluid, an increased percentage of neutrophils suggests a bacterial endocarditis.[25] Cytologic examination of pericardial fluid for the presence of malignant cells is an important part of the fluid analysis **(Color Plate 85)**. Decreased glucose levels are found with bacterial infections and malignancies. Gram stains and cultures are not routinely performed unless bacterial endocarditis is suspected. Pericardial fluid CEA levels show excellent correlation with cytologic studies.[41]

PERITONEAL FLUID

Accumulation of fluid in the peritoneal cavity is called ascites, and the fluid is commonly referred to as ascitic fluid rather than peritoneal fluid. Both transudates and exudates occur, and normal saline is sometimes introduced into the peritoneal cavity to act as a lavage for the detection of abdominal injuries that have not yet resulted in the accumulation of fluid. Analysis of lavage fluid is a particularly sensitive test for the detection of intra-abdominal bleeding.[26]

TABLE 8–9. Pleural Fluid Characteristics in Common Diseases*

ETIOLOGY	APPEARANCE	TOTAL WBC (per μl)	PREDOMINANT WBC	RBC (per μl)	PROTEIN	GLUCOSE	LDH	AMYLASE	pH
Transudates									
Congestive heart failure	Clear, straw-colored	< 1000	M	0–1000	PF/S < 0.5	PF = S	PF/S < 0.6 < 200 IU/liter	≤ S	> 7.40
Cirrhosis	Clear, straw-colored	< 500	M	< 1000	PF/S < 0.5	PF = S	PF/S < 0.6 < 200 IU/liter	≤ S	> 7.40
Exudates									
Parapneumonic (uncomplicated)	Turbid	5,000–25,000	P	< 5000	PF/S > 0.5	PF = S	PF/S > 0.6	≤ S	> 7.30
Empyema	Turbid to purulent	25,000–100,000	P	< 5000	PF/S > 0.5	0–60 mg/dl PF/S < 0.5	PF/S > 0.6 some > 1000 IU/liter	≤ S	< 7.30
Pulmonary infarction	Straw-colored to bloody	5,000–15,000	P	1,000–100,000	PF/S > 0.5	PF = S	PF/S > 0.6	≤ S	> 7.30
Tuberculosis	Straw-colored to serosanguineous	5,000–10,000	M	< 10,000	PF/S > 0.5	PF = S or < 60 mg/dl	PF/S > 0.6	≤ S	< or > 7.30
Rheumatoid disease	Turbid, green to yellow	1,000–20,000	M or P	< 1000	PF/S > 0.5	< 30 mg/dl	Often > 1000 IU/liter	≤ S	< 7.30
Carcinoma	Turbid to bloody	< 10,000	M	1,000 to several 100,000	PF/S > 0.5	PF = S or < 60 mg/dl	PF/S > 0.6	≤ S	< or > 7.30
Pancreatitis	Turbid	5,000–20,000	P	1,000–10,000	PFS > 0.5	PF = S	PF/S > 0.6	PF/S > 2	> 7.30

*From Sahn,[45] p 106–107, with permission.
WBC = white blood cells, RBC = red blood cells, LDH = lactic dehydrogenase, M = mononuclear, PF = pleural fluid, S = serum, IU = international units, P = polymorphonuclear.

Like pleural and pericardial fluids, normal peritoneal fluid is clear and pale yellow. Exudates are turbid with bacterial or fungal infections **(Color Plate 86)**, and may appear green when bile is present. The presence of bile can be confirmed using standard chemical screening tests for bilirubin, including urine reagent strips and ferric chloride spot tests. Chylous or pseudochylous material also may be present. Cellular examination may show macrophages with ingested fat **(Color Plate 87)**.

Normal red blood cell counts are usually below 100,000 cells per μl. Elevated counts may indicate hemorrhagic trauma. Should the fluid appear visually bloody, it may not be necessary to perform an actual count. Normal white blood cell counts are below 300 cells per μl, and the count increases with bacterial peritonitis and cirrhosis. To distinguish between those two conditions, an absolute granulocyte count should be performed. An absolute granulocyte count greater than 250 cells per cubic milliliter is indicative of infection.[27] Cytologic examination for malignant cells is, of course, a very important procedure **(Color Plates 88 and 89)**. The presence of psammoma bodies may be seen in benign conditions, but if they are accompanied by atypical cells, careful examination should be performed because they are frequently associated with ovarian and thyroid tumors **(Color Plate 90)**. Measurement of fluid CEA levels can provide valuable diagnostic information in malignancy.[1]

Chemical examination of ascitic fluid consists primarily of glucose, amylase, and alkaline phosphatase determinations. Glucose is decreased below serum levels in tubercular peritonitis and abnormal malignancy. Amylase is routinely determined on ascitic fluid to ascertain cases of pancreatitis, and it may also be elevated in gastrointestinal perforations. An elevated alkaline phosphatase is also highly diagnostic of intestinal perforation. Measurements of blood urea nitrogen and creatinine in the fluid are requested when there is concern about a ruptured bladder or accidental puncture of the bladder during the paracentesis.[15]

Gram stains and bacterial cultures for both aerobes and anaerobes are performed when bacterial peritonitis is suspected, and acid-fast stains and cultures for tuberculosis may also be requested.

SUMMARY OF SEROUS FLUID TESTING

Pleural Fluid

Normal appearance: Clear, pale yellow

Turbidity: White blood cells and microorganisms

Blood: Traumatic injury, malignancy, traumatic tap

Milky: Chylous or pseudochylous material

Sudan III: Chylous material

Neutrophils: Bacterial infection

Lymphocytes: Tuberculosis, malignancy

Normal glucose: Parallels serum glucose

Low glucose: Tuberculosis, rheumatoid inflammation, malignancy

Low pH: Tuberculosis, malignancy, esophageal rupture

Elevated amylase: Pancreatitis

CEA: Malignancy

Pericardial Fluid

Normal appearance: Clear, pale yellow

Milky: Lymphatic drainage

Turbidity: Infection, malignancy

Blood: Tuberculosis, tumor, cardiac puncture

Neutrophils: Bacterial endocarditis

Low glucose: Bacterial infection, malignrancy

CEA: Malignancy

Peritoneal Fluid

Normal appearance: Clear, pale yellow

Turbidity: Peritonitis, cirrhosis

Green: Bile

Milky: Chylous or pseudochylous material

Blood: Trauma

Neutrophils: Peritonitis

Low glucose: Tubercular peritonitis, malignancy

Elevated amylase: Pancreatitis, gastrointestinal perforation

Elevated alkaline phosphatase: Intestinal perforation

Elevated urea or creatinine: Ruptured bladder

AMNIOTIC FLUID

Although much of the current interest in amniotic fluid is in the field of cytogenetics, several very significant tests are performed in the routine clinical laboratory and are discussed in this section.

Amniotic fluid is found in the membranous sac that surrounds the fetus and provides a cushion to protect the fetus (Fig. 8–8). The fluid is formed from the metabolism of fetal cells, transfer of water across the placental membrane, and, in later stages of development, by fetal urine. However, by the time production of fetal urine occurs, the fetus begins swallowing the amniotic fluid in an amount approximately equal to the urine output. Therefore, the buildup of amniotic fluid to a total volume of 500 to 2500 ml at term is produced primarily by increased cell metabolism and placental water exchanges. Inability of the fetus to swallow is a critical sign and is indicated by an abnormal increase in amniotic fluid.[16]

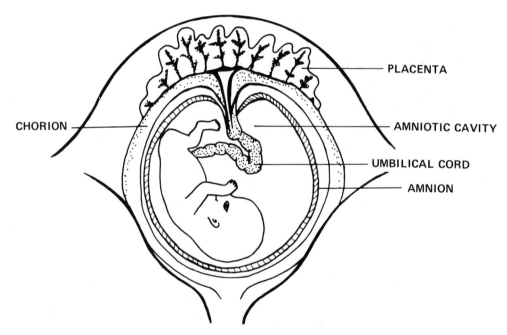

FIGURE 8–8. Fetus in amniotic sac.

Fluid for analysis is obtained by needle aspiration into the amniotic sac, a procedure called amniocentesis. The procedure is relatively safe and can be performed on an outpatient basis. Specimens should be protected from light and promptly delivered to the laboratory. Special precautions must be taken with specimens for cytogenetic analysis because cells in the fluid must be kept alive for culturing by the laboratory. A 20-ml fluid sample may contain as few as 10 cells! If cell culturing cannot be done immediately, the specimen should be incubated at 37°C for no longer than 2 days. Specimens that must be transported for analysis should be sent by express, courier-delivered mail to ensure prompt delivery. Cytogenetic analysis has become an important predictor of birth defects.

FETAL DISTRESS

Clinical analysis of amniotic fluid assesses both fetal well-being and maturation. Because amniotic fluid is a product of fetal metabolism, the constituents that are present in the fluid provide information about the metabolic processes taking place and the progress of fetal maturation. When conditions that adversely affect the fetus arise, the danger to the fetus must be measured against the ability of the fetus to survive an early delivery.

The oldest routinely performed laboratory test on amniotic fluid evaluates the severity of the fetal anemia produced by hemolytic disease of the newborn. In lay terms, these infants are referred to as "Rh babies." The incidence of this disease has been decreasing rapidly since the development of methods to prevent anti-Rh antibody production in postpartum mothers. However, the problem does and will continue to exist, so laboratory personnel must be prepared to analyze these specimens. The destruction of fetal red blood cells by antibodies that are present in the maternal circulation results in the appearance of the red blood cell degradation product, bilirubin, in the amniotic fluid. By measuring the amount of bilirubin present in the fluid, it is possible to determine the degree of hemolysis taking place and to assess the danger this anemia presents to the fetus.

The measurement of amniotic fluid bilirubin is performed by spectrophotometric analysis. As illustrated in Figure 8–9, the optical density of the fluid is measured in intervals between 365 mμ and 550 mμ, and the readings are plotted on semilogarithmic graph paper. In normal fluid, the optical density will be highest at 365 mμ and will decrease linearly (Plot A) to 550 mμ. However, when bilirubin is present, a rise in optical density will be seen at 450 mμ because this is the wave length of maximum bilirubin absorption (Plot B). The amount of bilirubin present can be determined from the height of the peak, thereby providing a measure of the degree of red cell destruction. Extreme care must be taken to protect the specimen from light, because bilirubin is a very light-sensitive chemical and markedly decreased values will be obtained with as little as 30 minutes of exposure to light.[16]

In cases of premature or prolonged rupture of the amniotic membranes there is concern over possible infection of the mother and fetus. Testing of the fluid with the leukocyte esterase reagent strip for the presence of white blood cells has recently been shown to be a good indicator of infection and is more rapid and cost effective than Gram stains and cultures.[22]

FETAL MATURITY

Fetal distress, whether caused by hemolytic disease of the newborn or other conditions, forces the obstetrician to consider a preterm delivery. At this point, it becomes necessary to assess fetal maturity. Respiratory distress is the most frequent complication of early delivery. Therefore, laboratory tests are performed to determine the maturity of the fetal lung, as well as the overall fetal maturity.

The laboratory procedure routinely used to measure fetal lung maturity is the lecithin-sphingomyelin ratio (L/S ratio). Lecithin is the primary component of the phospholipids that make up the majority of the alveolar lining and account for alveolar stability.

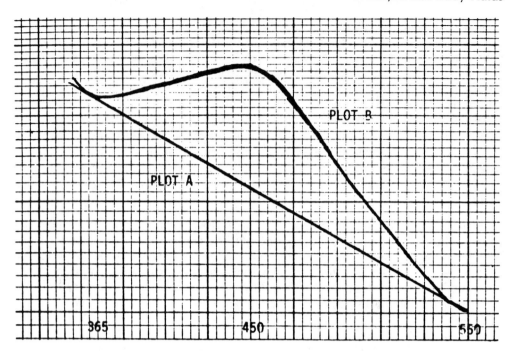

FIGURE 8–9. Spectrophotometric amniotic fluid bilirubin scans.

Lecithin is produced at a relatively low and constant rate until the 35th week of gestation, at which time a noticeable increase in its production occurs, resulting in the stabilization of the fetal lung alveoli. Sphingomyelin is a lipid that is produced at a constant rate throughout fetal gestation; therefore, it can serve as a control on which to base the rise in lecithin. Both lecithin and sphingomyelin appear in the amniotic fluid in amounts proportional to their concentrations in the fetus.[17] Prior to 35 weeks of gestation, the L/S ratio is usually less than 1.6, and it will rise to 2.0 or higher when lecithin production increases. Therefore, when the L/S ratio reaches 2.0 a preterm delivery is usually considered to be a relatively safe procedure.[58] Measurement of lecithin and sphingomyelin is performed using thin-layer chromatography.[38]

Although the L/S ratio is considered the standard fetal maturity test, there are some complications, including the equipment and time needed to perform thin-layer chromatography; interference in amniotic fluid contaminated by blood, meconium, and vaginal mucus; and the inability to detect another essential lung surface lipid, phosphatidylglycerol. Absence of phosphatidylglycerol in the presence of a normal L/S ratio is seen in children of diabetic mothers; and even though phosphatidylglycerol represents only 10 percent of the lung surface lipids, respiratory distress will occur if it is present.[18] Therefore, demonstration of phosphatidylglycerol on a thin-layer chromatograph has usually been included in the testing for fetal lung maturity. Analysis of phosphatidylglycerol is not compromised by amniotic fluid contamination. Some laboratories perform a lung profile in which concentrations of lecithin, sphingomyelin, phosphatidylglycerol, phosphatidylinositol, and other lung surface lipids are measured.[3] No correlation between the presence or absence of phosphatidylinositol and the occurrence of respiratory distress has been demonstrated.[52] However, because the appearance of phosphatidylinositol in amniotic fluid parallels that of lecithin, measurement of phosphatidylglycerol and phosphatidylinositol may be used in place of the L/S ratio when fluid is contaminated.[19]

Development of an immunologic agglutination test for phosphatidylglycerol has provided a more rapid method for assessment of fetal maturity that does not require a laboratory to be equipped to perform thin-layer chromatography. The Aminostat-FLM (Hana Biologic, Inc., Berkeley, CA) utilizes antisera specific for phosphatidylglycerol and is not

TABLE 8–10. Tests for Fetal Well-being and Maturity

TEST	NORMAL VALUES AT TERM[16]	SIGNIFICANCE
Bilirubin scan	0.025 mg/dl	Hemolytic disease of the newborn
L/S ratio	2.0	Fetal lung maturity
Phosphatidylglycerol	Present	Fetal lung maturity
Foam stability index	>47	Fetal lung maturity
Creatinine	1.8–4.0 mg/dl	Fetal age
Alpha fetal protein	4.0 mg/dl	Neural tube disorders

affected by specimen contamination. Studies have shown good correlation with thin-layer chromatography but with a slightly higher incidence of false-negatives that may need to be followed up with further testing.[6][44]

Until the development of biochemical techniques to measure the individual lung surface lipid concentrations, a mechanical screening test, called the "foam" or "shake" test, was used to determine their presence. Because it can be performed at the bedside or in the laboratory, the test is still in use. Amniotic fluid is mixed with 95 percent ethanol, shaken for 15 seconds, and then allowed to sit undisturbed for 15 minutes. At the end of this time, the surface of the fluid is observed for the presence of a continuous line of bubbles around the outside edge. The presence of bubbles correlates well with fetal lung maturity, although the analysis is more subjective than the L/S ratio.[10]

A modification of the foam test uses 0.5 ml of amniotic fluid added to varying amounts of 95 percent ethanol, providing a gradient of ethanol/fluid ratios ranging from 0.44 to 0.50 in 0.01 increments which can be used to provide a semiquantitative measure of the amount of surface lipid present. A value of 47 or higher indicates fetal lung maturity. The Foam Stability Index has shown good correlation with the L/S ratio and phosphatidylglycerol test and provides a rapid, low-cost means for assessing fetal lung maturity.[50] The test is available in kit form using cassettes of measured ethanol combined with an inert blue dye for better visualization (Lumadex-FSI, Beckman Instruments, Inc., Brea, CA).

Fetal age can be determined by measuring the amount of creatinine in the amniotic fluid. At about 36 weeks of gestation, urine from the fetal kidney begins appearing in the amniotic fluid; therefore, a creatinine concentration above 2.0 mg per dl indicates a fetal age of approximately 36 weeks.[57] As more is learned about the role of the fetal metabolites that are present in the amniotic fluid in the assessment of fetal well-being and maturity, additional chemical tests will become part of the amniotic fluid analysis. Already, the measurement of alpha fetal protein levels and acetylcholinesterase activity is being used to provide early detection of neural tube disorders, such as spina bifida and anencephaly.[2] Table 8–10 summarizes the routine chemical tests performed on amniotic fluid.

SWEAT

Although the analysis of sweat is not a frequently requested clinical laboratory procedure, measurement of the sweat electrolytes, sodium and chloride, is performed to confirm the diagnosis of cystic fibrosis. Cystic fibrosis is a metabolic disease that affects the mucus-secreting glands of the body. It is inherited as an autosomal recessive and is seen in approximately 1 out of every 1500 to 2000 Caucasian births.[55] Because cystic fibrosis involves multiple organs, many clinical symptoms can lead the physician to suspect its presence. The most common indicators include family history of cystic fibrosis, newborns who fail to thrive or who have intestinal obstructions, and the appearance of pancreatic insufficiency or respiratory distress in infants. The demonstration of elevated sweat sodium and chloride values in patients who exhibit any or all of these symptoms serves to confirm the diagnosis of cystic fibrosis.

Proper collection and handling of sweat specimens can present a problem for the laboratory when one considers that the patient, often an infant, must be induced to sweat and that the sweat produced cannot be aspirated into a collection tube. Earlier methods to stimulate the production of sweat, including the use of humid, high-temperature rooms and encasing the patient's body in plastic, were replaced by Gibson and Cooke's[51] pilocarpine iontophoresis technique. Sweat glands on the forearm are subjected to the sweat-inducing alkaloid pilocarpine in the presence of a mild electrical current. Following stimulation, the area is thoroughly cleansed, and preweighed electrolyte-free gauze or filter paper is placed with the use of forceps on the stimulated area and tightly sealed to prevent evaporation. Using pilocarpine iontophoresis, a sufficient amount of sweat for analysis can be collected in 25 to 30 minutes. After reweighing the pads to determine the amount of sweat collected, the sweat is eluted using a measured amount of deionized water.

Chloride is measured by automatic or manual titration methods and sodium by flame photometry or ion-exchange electrodes. Sweat chloride and sodium values over 70 mEq per liter are seen consistently in 98 percent of patients with cystic fibrosis and are almost never found in normal individuals. Concentrations over 40 mEq per liter are considered borderline, and the test should be repeated at a later date if the patient's clinical symptoms so warrant.[5]

The actual collection of sweat can be avoided by applying a chloride electrode to the skin following stimulation and measuring the concentration directly. However, because the amount of sodium present should approximate the chloride concentration, most laboratories prefer to measure both parameters to provide better quality control of the procedure.[55] The method may also produce inaccurate readings in the high ranges when influenced by air bubbles and temperature fluctuations.[56]

Recently, comparisons between sweat electrolytes and sweat osmolarity have shown good correlation. After pilocarpine iontophoresis stimulation, a vapor pressure osmometer pad is placed directly on the surface and sealed with plastic. Because the sweat osmolarity is measured on an undiluted sample, care must be taken to include the water that condenses on the plastic cover or values will be falsely elevated.[56] A collection system (Model 3500, Webster Sweat Collection System, Wescor, Logan, UT) eliminates the condensation error by the use of a heated collection cup on the osmometer pad.

Use of the osmometer method for measuring sweat electrolytes provides a means for evaluation of young infants without subjecting them to the rigors of traditional sweat collection methods. The test should be performed on infants older than 8 days, because newborn infants consistently have high electrolyte concentrations. Early diagnosis of cystic fibrosis is essential for prolonged patient survival. An osmolarity reading greater than 210 mmol/kg is indicative of cystic fibrosis, and a reading less than 170 mmol/kg is considered normal. Borderline values should be reevaluated, and positive results should be followed later with sweat electrolyte testing.[49]

REFERENCES

1. Berti, P, et al: Diagnostic values of glycoproteins, immunoglobulin, complement and CEA in pleural and peritoneal effusions. Quad Sclavo Diagn 17(4):483–494, 1981.

2. Brock, DJH: Prenatal diagnosis: Chemical methods. Br Med Bull 31(1):16–19, 1976.

3. Broderick, PA, et al: Exfoliative cytology: Interpretation of synovial fluid in disease. J Bone Joint Surg 58-A(3):396–399, 1976.

4. Bunch, TW, et al: Synovial fluid complement determination as a diagnostic aid in inflammatory joint disease. Mayo Clin Proc 49:715–720, 1974.

5. Cannon, DC: Examination of the seminal fluid. In Henry, JB (ed): Clinical Diagnosis and Management by Laboratory Methods. WB Saunders, Philadelphia, 1984.

6. Chapman, JF: Current methods for evaluating fetal lung maturity. Lab Med 17(10):597–602, 1986.

7. Curtis, G, Newman, R, and Clack, M: Synovial fluid lactate and the diagnosis of septic arthritis. J Infect 6:239–246,1983.

8. Czuppon, AB and Mettler, I: Estimation of anti-spermatozoa antibody concentrations by a ^{125}I protein-A binding assay in sera of infertile patients. J Clin Chem Clin Biochem 21(6):357–362, 1983.

9. Dieppe, P, et al: Laboratory handling of crystals. Ann Rheum Dis (Suppl) 42:60–63, 1983.

10. Dover, JS and Elliet, HC: Unidimensional chromatographic determination of phosphatidyl glycerol and L/S ratio with predictive values of L/S ratio, phosphatidyl glycerol and foam stability index. Lab Med 13(3):159–161,1982.

11. Fraser, RG and Pare, JAP: Diagnosis of Disease of the Chest, Vol 1. WB Saunders, Philadelphia, 1977.

12. Fraysier, HD: A rapid screening technique for the detection of spermatozoa. J Forensic Sci 32(2):527–528, 1987.

13. Glasser, L: Seminal fluid and subfertility. Diagn Med 4(5):28–45, 1981.

14. Glasser, L: Body fluid analysis: Synovial fluid. Diagn Med 3(4):35–50, 1980.

15. Glasser, L: Body fluid evaluation: Serous fluids. Diagn Med 3(5):79–90, 1980.

16. Glasser, L: Amniotic fluid and the quality of life. Diagn Med 4(6):31–51, 1981.

17. Gluck, et al: Diagnosis of the respiratory distress syndrome by amniocentesis. Am J Obst Gynecol 109(3):440–445, 1971.

18. Hallman, M, et al: Absence of phosphatidylglycerol (PG) in respiratory distress syndrome in the newborn. Pediatr Res 11(6):714–720, 1977.

19. Hallman, M, et al: Phosphatidylinositol and phosphatidylglycerol in amniotic fluid: Indices of lung maturity. Am J Obstet Gynecol 125(5):613–617, 1976.

20. Hasselbacher, P: Variation in synovial fluid analysis by hospital laboratories. Arthritis Rheum 30(6):637–642, 1987.

21. Hernandez, OG, et al: Very low glucose concentrations in hypocellular malignant pleural effusions. So Med J 81(2):289, 1988.

22. Hoskins, IA, Johnson, TRB, and Winkle, CA: Leukocyte esterase activity in human amniotic fluid for the rapid detection of chorioamnionitis. Am J Obstet Gynecol 157(3):730–732, 1987.

23. Houston, MC: Pleural fluid pH: Diagnostic, therapeutic and prognostic value. Am J Surg 154(3):333–337,1987.

24. Jain, AP, Gupta, OP, and Khan, N: Comparative diagnostic efficiency of criteria used for differentiating transdudate and exudate pleural effusions. J Assoc Physicians India 30(11):823–825,1982.

25. Jay, SJ: Pleural effusions: Definitive evaluation of the exudate. Postgrad Med 80(5):181–188, 1986.

26. Jergens, ME: Peritoneal lavage. Am J Surg 133:365–369, 1977.

27. Jones, SR: The absolute granulocyte count in ascites fluid: An aid to the diagnosis of spontaneous bacterial peritonitis. West J Med 126(5):344–346, 1977.

28. Keel, BS: The semen analysis: An important diagnostic evaluation. Lab Med 10(11):686–688, 1979.

29. Kjeldsberg, CR and Knight, JA: Body Fluids: Laboratory Examination of Amniotic Cerebrospinal, Seminal, Serous and Synovial Fluids: A Textbook Atlas. American Society of Clinical Pathologists, Chicago, 1986.

30. Kjeldsberg, CR and Krieg, A: Cerebrospinal fluid and other body fluids. In Henry, JB (ed): Clinical Diagnosis and Management by Laboratory Methods. WB Saunders, Philadelphia, 1984.

31. Kulovich, MV, Hallman, MB, and Gluck, L: The lung profile: Normal pregnancy. Am J Obstet Gynecol 135:57–60, 1979.

32. Light, R, et al: Pleural effusions: The diagnostic separation of transudates and exudates. Ann Intern Med 77:507–513,1971.

33. Light, RW, Erozan, YS, and Ball, WC: Cells in pleural fluid: Their value in differential diagnosis. Arch Intern Med 132:854–860, 1973.

34. Lopez, A, et al: Suitability of solid-phase chemistry for quantification of leukocytes in cerebrospinal, seminal and peritoneal fluid. Clin Chem 33(8):1475–1476, 1987.

35. Naib, ZM: Cytology of synovial fluids. Acta Cytol 17(4):299–309, 1973.

36. Ochi, T, Yonemasu, K, and Ono, K: Immunochemical quantitation of complement components of C1q and C3 in sera and synovial fluid of patients with bone and joint diseases. Ann Rheum Dis 39(3):235–240, 1980.

37. Overstreet, JW and Katz, DF: Semen analysis. Urol Clin North Am 14(3):441–449, 1987.

38. Pappas, AA, Mullins, RE, and Gadsden, RH: Improved one-dimensional thin-layer chromatography of phospholipids in amniotic fluid. Clin Chem 28(1):209–211, 1982.

39. Pekin, RJ, Malinin, TI, and Zvaiflen, NJ: Unusual synovial fluid findings in Reiter's syndrome. Ann Intern Med 66(4):677–684, 1967.

40. Phelps, P, Steele, AD, and McCarty, DJ: Compensated polarized light microscopy: Identification of crystals in synovial fluid from gout and pseudogout. JAMA 203(7):166–171, 1968.

41. Pinto, MM: Carcinoembryonic antigen in pericardial effusion. Lab Med 18(10):671–672, 1987.

42. Revill, PA: Examination of synovial fluid. Curr Top Pathol 71:2–24, 1982.

43. Rippey, J: Synovial fluid analysis. Lab Med 10(3):140–145, 1979.

44. Saad, SA, et al: The reliability and clinical use of a rapid phosphatidylglycerol assay in normal and diabetic pregnancies. Am J Obstet Gynecol 157(6):1516–1520, 1987.

45. Sahn, SA: Pulmonary diseases. In Reller, LB, Sahn, SA, and Schrier, RW (eds): Clinical Internal Medicine. Little, Brown & Co, Boston, 1979.

46. Sahn, SA: The differential diagnosis of pleural effusions. West J Med 137(2):99–108, 1982.

47. Sampson, JH and Alexander, NJ: Semen analysis: A laboratory approach. Lab Med 13(4):218–223, 1982.

48. Samuelson, CO and Ward, JR: Examination of the synovial fluid. J Fam Pract 14(2):343–349, 1982.

49. Schoni, MH, et al: Early diagnosis of cystic fibrosis by means of sweat microosmometry. J Pediatr 104(5):691,1984.

50. Sher, G, Statland, BE, and Freer, DE: Clinical evaluation of the quantitative foam stability index test. Obstet Gynecol 55:617–620, 1984.

51. Schwachman, H and Mahmoodian, A: The sweat test and cystic fibrosis. Diagn Med 5(4):61–77, 1982.

52. Skjaeraasen, J and Stray-Pedersen, S: Amniotic fluid phosphatidylinositol and phosphatidylglycerol: Normal pregnancy. Acta Obstet Gynecol Scand 58:225–229, 1979.

53. Strickland, DM and Ziaya, PR: Reduced sperm motility in plastic containers. Lab Med 18(5):310–312, 1987.

54. Teloh, HA: Clinical pathology of synovial fluid. Ann Clin Lab Sci 5(4):282–287, 1975.

55. Tocci, PM and McKey, RM: Laboratory confirmation of the diagnosis of cystic fibrosis. Clin Chem 22(11):1841–1844, 1976.
56. Webster, HL: Laboratory diagnosis of cystic fibrosis. CRC Crit Rev Clin Lab Sci 18(4):313–337, 1983.
57. Weiss, RR, et al: Amniotic fluid uric acid and creatinine as measures of fetal maturity. Obstet Gynecol 44(2):208–214, 1974.
58. Went, RE, Rosenbaum, J and Statland, BE: Amniotic fluid and antenatal diagnosis. In Henry, JB (ed): Clinical Diagnosis and Management by Laboratory Methods. WB Saunders, Philadelphia, 1984.

STUDY QUESTIONS (Choose one best answer)

1. Proper collection of a semen specimen should include all of the following except
   a. collection in a sterile container
   b. collection after a 3-day period of sexual abstinence
   c. collection at the laboratory followed by 1 hour of refrigeration
   d. collection at home and delivery to the laboratory within 1 hour

2. Semen specimens should be analyzed
   a. immediately upon receipt
   b. prior to liquefaction
   c. after liquefaction
   d. one hour after collection

3. An abnormal amount of prostatic fluid in a semen specimen will
   a. lower the pH
   b. raise the pH
   c. increase the viscosity
   d. decrease the viscosity

4. The normal sperm count is
   a. 140 to 200 million per milliliter
   b. 50 to 100 million per microliter
   c. 20 to 160 million per milliliter
   d. 50 to 100 million per microliter

5. The purpose of diluting semen specimens with sodium bicarbonate and formalin prior to counting is to
   a. ensure liquefaction of the specimen
   b. allow motility to be determined while performing the count
   c. enhance the cellular morphology
   d. immobilize and preserve the sperm

6. The motility component of a sperm analysis includes all of the following except
   a. differentiation between progressive and brownian movement
   b. determination of the percentage of motile sperm
   c. determination of the quality of movement
   d. differentiation between motility of normal and abnormal sperm

7. An acceptable percentage of abnormal sperm after examination of 200 cells is
   a. zero
   b. less than 10%
   c. less than 30%
   d. less than 50%

8. A normal semen analysis followed by continued infertility may be the result of
   a. decreased concentration of fructose
   b. decreased sperm viability
   c. sperm agglutinins in the male
   d. sperm agglutinins in the female

9. Semen analysis on post-vasectomy patients should be performed
   a. within 1 week
   b. one month post-vasectomy
   c. until two consecutive monthly specimens show no sperm
   d. until two consecutive monthly specimens show no viable sperm

10. The presence or absence of semen in a specimen can accurately be determined by testing for
    a. fructose
    b. alkaline phosphatase
    c. acid phosphatase
    d. agglutinating antibodies

11. All of the following statements on synovial fluid are true except
    a. it surrounds all joints in the body
    b. it is found only in the knee
    c. it acts as a lubricant
    d. it supplies nourishment to cartilage

12. Which of the following descriptions of synovial fluid does not match
    a. normal = clear, pale yellow
    b. crystals = milky
    c. traumatic tap = blood streaks
    d. sepsis = uniform blood

13. In the Ropes, or mucin clot, test, normal synovial fluid
    a. forms a solid clot when added to hydrochloric acid
    b. forms a solid clot when added to glacial acetic acid
    c. forms a friable clot when added to hydrochloric acid
    d. forms a friable clot when added to glacial acetic acid

14. A white blood cell count on synovial fluid obtained during a traumatic tap should be diluted with
    a. glacial acetic acid and methylene blue
    b. 0.1N hydrochloric acid and methylene blue
    c. normal saline and methylene blue
    d. hypotonic saline and methylene blue

15. Neutrophils that contain precipitated rheumatoid factor in their cytoplasm are called
    a. LE cells
    b. Reiter cells
    c. ragocytes
    d. macrophages

16. Synovial fluid for crystal examination should be
    a. stained with Wright's stain and examined with bright-field microscopy
    b. stained with methylene blue and examined under polarized light
    c. examined unstained under direct and compensated polarized light
    d. examined unstained with bright-field microscopy

17. Crystals found in synovial fluid during attacks of gout are
    a. monosodium urate
    b. calcium pyrophosphate
    c. cholesterol
    d. apatite

18. Examination of synovial fluid under direct polarized light reveals intracellular needle-shaped crystals that appear white against the black background. When a red compensator is added and the crystals are aligned with the slow vibration, they appear yellow against the red background. These crystals are
    a. monosodium urate showing positive birefringence
    b. monosodium urate showing negative birefringence
    c. calcium pyrophosphate showing positive birefringence
    d. calcium pyrophosphate showing negative birefringence

19. Crystals that appear as rhombic-shaped or as needle-shaped and are blue when aligned with the slow vibration of compensated polarized light are
    a. monosodium urate
    b. calcium pyrophosphate
    c. apatite
    d. corticosteroid

20. In gout, both serum and synovial fluid will have increased levels of
    a. glucose
    b. protein
    c. uric acid
    d. complement

21. A cloudy, yellow-green synovial fluid with 100,000 WBCs, a predominance of neutrophils, and a decreased glucose would be classified as
    a. noninflammatory
    b. inflammatory
    c. septic
    d. crystal-induced

22. An arthrocentesis performed on a patient with lupus erythematosus produces a cloudy yellow fluid with 2000 WBCs, of which 55% are neutrophils. This fluid would be classified as
    a. noninflammatory
    b. inflammatory
    c. septic
    d. crystal-induced

23. Fluid collected by thoracentesis is called
    a. pleural
    b. pericardial
    c. peritoneal
    d. ascitic

24. Serous fluid effusions may result from all of the following except
    a. congestive heart failure
    b. hypoalbuminemia
    c. increased capillary permeability
    d. dehydration

25. Effusions produced by conditions that directly affect the serous membranes are termed

    a. transudates
    b. exudates

26. To be classified as an exudate, a fluid should have

    a. total protein less than 3 g/dl, specific gravity less than 1.015, and LD less than 200 IU
    b. total protein less than 3 g/dl, specific gravity greater than 1.015, and LD greater than 200 IU
    c. total protein greater than 3 g/dl, specific gravity greater than 1.015, and LD greater than 200 IU
    d. total protein greater than 3 g/dl, cell count less than 1000/μl, and fluid to serum LD ratio less than 0.6

27. Differentiation between a hemothorax and a hemorrhagic exudate on a bloody pleural fluid is done by

    a. observing the fluid for streaks of blood, because this indicates a hemothorax
    b. performing a hematocrit, because a hemothorax will give a value similar to the whole blood
    c. performing an RBC count, because a hemorrhagic effusion will have a count over 100,000/μl
    d. performing both RBC and WBC counts, because a hemothorax will have marked elevations of both cell types

28. A milky pleural fluid becomes clear after extraction with ether. This fluid contained

    a. chylous material from thoracic duct leakage
    b. pseudochylous material from thoracic duct leakage
    c. chylous material from inflammation
    d. pseudochylous material from inflammation

29. A pleural fluid pH of less than 6.0 is indicative of

    a. tuberculosis
    b. malignancy
    c. pancreatic disorders
    d. esophageal rupture

30. Peritoneal lavage is performed to

    a. remove ascitic fluid
    b. check for the presence of bile
    c. detect intra-abdominal bleeding
    d. provide a sufficient volume of fluid for chemical analysis

31. Requests for amylase and alkaline phosphatase determinations on ascitic fluid are received in suspected cases of

    a. peritonitis
    b. gastrointestinal perforations
    c. ruptured bladder
    d. malignancy

32. Amniotic fluid is formed by all of the following except

    a. fetal urine
    b. fetal cell metabolism
    c. fetal swallowing
    d. transfer of water across the placenta

33. An amniocentesis is performed on a woman whose last two pregnancies have resulted in stillbirths due to hemolytic disease of the newborn. A screening test performed at the hospital is positive for bilirubin, and the specimen is sent to a reference lab for a bilirubin scan. Doctors are concerned when the report comes back negative, and they question if

    a. the correct specimen was sent
    b. the specimen was refrigerated
    c. the specimen was exposed to light
    d. the specimen reached the reference lab within 30 minutes

34. Tests to determine the maturity of the fetal lung and overall fetal maturity are

    a. bilirubin, L/S ratio, and creatinine
    b. bilirubin, L/S ratio, and phosphatidylglycerol
    c. creatinine, L/S ratio, and phosphatidylglycerol
    d. L/S ratio and phosphatidylglycerol

35. The foam, or shake, test is a screening test for amniotic fluid

    a. bilirubin
    b. L/S ratio
    c. alpha fetal protein
    d. phosphatidylglycerol

36. Sweat electrolytes run on specimens collected by pilocarpine iontophoresis are

    a. elevated in muscular dystrophy
    b. elevated in cystic fibrosis
    c. decreased in cystic fibrosis
    d. decreased in muscular dystrophy

GASTRIC ANALYSIS

LEARNING OBJECTIVES

Upon completion of this chapter, the reader will be able to

1. describe the production and composition of the gastric secretion
2. differentiate between total acidity and titratable acidity
3. calculate the milliequivalents per liter of titratable acid when provided with the appropriate titration data
4. calculate the acid output, maximum acid output, and peak acid output when provided with the appropriate titration data
5. state the normal volume, acid output, and significance of the basal gastric analysis
6. discuss the advantages and disadvantages of the pentagastrin, histamine, Histalog, and insulin stimulation tests
7. describe the typical poststimulation gastric analysis results in hyperacidity and pernicious anemia
8. define anacidity

Due to the development of nonlaboratory procedures for the evaluation of gastric function which are considered more precise, less time consuming, and less uncomfortable for the patient, routine examination of gastric contents by the clinical laboratory has been diminishing. Of major interest in the laboratory analysis of gastric secretion is the measurement of gastric acidity, which has been considered useful in the diagnosis and treatment of peptic ulcers, pernicious anemia, Zollinger-Ellison syndrome, and the monitoring of surgical procedures. Additional procedures now in use for the detection of these disorders include direct examination of lesions by endoscopy, improved radiologic techniques, pH-sensitive electrodes that will transmit pH readings when passed into the stomach, measurement of serum gastrin levels, cytologic examination of gastric contents for malignant cells, and immunologic testing of serum for the presence of anti-intrinsic factor and antiparietal cell antibodies seen in pernicious anemia.[1] The sophistication of these procedures has reduced the diagnostic role of actual gastric acidity titration to a secondary one in many instances. However, inasmuch as the analysis is still requested by some physicians, students should be instructed in the performance and significance of the procedure and its relationship to other examinations currently being utilized.

PHYSIOLOGY

Gastric acidity results from the secretion of hydrochloric acid by the parietal cells in the stomach. These cells are also responsible for the production of intrinsic factor necessary for the intestinal absorption of vitamin B_{12}. Hydrochloric acid converts the enzyme precursor pepsinogen, secreted by the zymogen chief cells, to the enzyme pepsin, which catalyzes the digestion of protein. Stimulation of the parietal cells to produce acid is caused primarily by the hormone gastrin, which is secreted by specialized G cells in the lower portion of the stomach. Neurologic stimulation by the vagus nerve and the presence of food and fluid in the stomach promote the G cells to secrete gastrin. Besides the two major components, hydrochloric acid and pepsin, gastric secretions may also contain saliva, mucus, acid-neutralizing chemicals, and material regurgitated from intestinal, biliary, and pancreatic secretions.

SPECIMEN COLLECTION

Gastric contents are collected by nasal or oral intubation of the patient. To ensure complete collection of gastric secretions, the position of the tube is checked by fluoroscopic examination of the stomach. Patients should be instructed not to swallow excessive amounts of saliva during the collection period, because saliva will neutralize the gastric acidity. Collection is usually performed on patients in the fasting state. A more complete recovery of the gastric contents is obtained if aspiration is performed continuously throughout the collection period. However, because acidity testing is routinely performed on 15-minute specimens, the aspiration must be collected in time-labeled containers that represent each 15 minutes of the required collection period, and not as a single specimen.

OLD TITRATION PROCEDURES

Routine tests performed on gastric specimens include volume, pH, and titratable acidity. Different theories have existed concerning the types of acids present and their significance in the disease process. For many years, it was believed that acid with a pH less than 3.5 represented "free" or hydrochloric acid, and that the remainder of the acid present below pH 8.4 was "combined" or organic acid. The two acids were measured separately by titrating the specimen first with 0.1N NaOH, using the indicator Töpfer's reagent, which changes from red to yellow at pH 3.5. Then the titration was continued using phenolphthalein as an indicator and titrating from colorless to a faint pink color that appears at approximately pH 8.4. The titration using Töpfer's reagent represented the hydrochloric acid present; the titration with phenolphthalein measured the organic acid. The sum of the two titrations determined the total acidity of the specimen. The results were reported in "degrees of acidity," which represented the number of milliliters of 0.1N NaOH that were needed to titrate 100 ml of gastric secretion to the end point of the indicator being used (3.5 with Töpfer's reagent, and 8.4 with phenolphthalein).[3]

CURRENT TITRATION PROCEDURE

Current theories question the existence of two distinct gastric acid phases and recommend the measurement of the overall hydrogen ion concentration. Therefore, both the ionized and un-ionized hydrogen are measured simultaneously by titrating the specimen with 0.1N NaOH to pH 7.0 using the indicator phenol red, which changes from yellow to red in the pH range 6.6 to 8.0. Titration results are reported as milliequivalents or millimoles per liter of titratable acid, rather than in "degrees of acidity." This is a more conventional manner of test reporting, although, as can be seen from the definition of "degrees of acidity," the numerical results will be the same. Milliequivalents per liter of titratable acid are calculated from the amount of 0.1N NaOH needed to reach the phenol red end point using the standard formula $C_1 \times V_1 = C_2 \times V_2$.

Example: Calculate the milliequivalents per liter of titratable acid in a 20-ml specimen when 2.0 ml of 0.1N NaOH are used to reach pH 7.0.

$$0.1N \text{ NaOH} \times 2 \text{ ml} = X \times 20 \text{ ml}$$
$$20X = 0.2$$
$$X = 0.01 \text{ equivalents/liter}$$
$$0.01 \text{ equivalents/liter} \times 1000 = 10 \text{ mEq/liter}$$

Notice that when 0.1N is used in the calculation, the answer is in equivalents per liter and must be changed to milliequivalents per liter by multiplying by 1000. This can be avoided by converting the 0.1N NaOH to 100 mEq or 100 mmole prior to performing the calculation.

Because titratable acidity represents the milliequivalents or millimoles of acid per liter, and the typical gastric secretion specimen is of considerably less volume, it also becomes necessary to calculate the actual acid output in the specimen. This is done by multiplying the specimen volume in liters by the titratable acidity.

Example: The first 15-minute specimen of a 1-hour basal collection has a volume of 25 ml. To titrate 10 ml of this specimen to the end point of phenol red, 5 ml of 0.1N NaOH are used. Calculate the titratable acidity and the acid output of the specimen.

A. $100 \text{ mEq/liter NaOH} \times 5 \text{ ml} = X \times 10 \text{ ml}$
   $10X = 500 \text{ mEq/liter}$
   $X = 50 \text{ mEq/liter titratable acid}$

B. $\dfrac{25 \text{ ml specimen}}{1000 \text{ ml}} \times 50 \text{ mEq/liter} = 1.25 \text{ mEq acid/specimen}$

BASAL GASTRIC ACIDITY

The above example refers to the basal, or fasting, specimen, which is the initial collection in the gastric analysis. The basal specimen is a 1-hour collection, usually consisting of four 15-minute specimens, although any other time frame may be used, including a single 1-hour collection. The volume, pH, titratable acidity, and acid output of the samples that constitute the basal specimen are determined. Normal values for volume and acidity are based on the total 1-hour specimen. Therefore, individual sample results must be combined to provide the 1-hour total. A wide variety of normal values for the basal gastric secretion can be found throughout the literature; however, in general, the normal basal secretion has a volume of about 30 to 60 ml and contains a low acid output of approximately 1.0 to 4.0 mEq per hour.[1] Besides providing a baseline upon which to compare subsequent test results, the major diagnostic value of the basal gastric analysis lies in the finding of markedly elevated acidity. This is indicative of the Zollinger-Ellison syndrome, a condition of gastric hypersecretion produced by a gastrin-secreting tumor of the pancreas.

POSTSTIMULATION GASTRIC ACIDITY

The inability to produce gastric acidity cannot be determined solely from the analysis of the basal gastric secretion; therefore, additional tests must be performed. Several test variations are available, but all utilize the same principle, which is to introduce a gastric stimulant into the patient following the basal collection. Specimens continue to be collected and are tested for increased volume and acid content. Commonly used stimulants include pentagastrin, histamine, and Histalog. The stimulant of choice is currently pentagastrin, a synthetic compound resembling gastrin, because it does not cause the patient the discomfort that occurs with histamine administration, and it produces a more rapid

TABLE 9–1. Sample Gastric Analysis*

SPECIMEN #		SPECIMEN VOLUME	VOLUME TITRATED	M1 0.1N NaOH USED	TITRATABLE ACIDITY (mEq/liter)	ACID OUTPUT (mEq)	BASAL ACID OUTPUT (mEq/hr)	MAXIMUM ACID OUTPUT (mEq/hr)	PEAK ACID OUTPUT (mEq/hr)
Basal	#1	10	10	2.2	22	0.22			
	#2	15	10	2.0	20	0.30			
	#3	20	10	1.5	15	0.30			
	#4	5	5	2.5	50	0.25	1.07		
Stimulated	#1	30	10	6.5	65	1.95			
	#2	50	10	12.5	125	6.25			Times 2 = 25.5
	#3	50	10	13.0	130	6.50			
	#4	40	10	11.5	115	4.60		19.3	

*Analysis of four 15-minute basal specimens and four 15-minute specimens collected following administration of pentagastrin.

TABLE 9–2. Representative Normal and Abnormal Gastric Analysis Results[1, 4]

	BASAL ACID OUTPUT (mEq/hr)	MAXIMUM ACID OUTPUT (mEq/hr)	BAO/MAO
Normal	2.5	25.0	10%
Pernicious anemia	0	0	0
Duodenal ulcer	5.0	30.0	17%
Zollinger-Ellison syndrome	18.0	25.0	72%

response than Histalog. When pentagastrin or histamine is utilized as the stimulant, specimens are collected at 15-minute intervals for 1 hour following the injection. When Histalog is administered, the collection must continue for 2 hours because maximum acid output is delayed. A 2-hour collection of both basal and poststimulation samples is required when performing the insulin hypoglycemia test used to determine whether surgical removal of the vagus nerve has been successful. Insulin stimulation of the parietal cells to produce acid is transmitted by the vagus nerve; therefore, following a successful vagotomy postinsulin stimulation gastric acidity will be no greater than basal acidity.[2]

All poststimulation specimens are analyzed in the same manner as the basal specimens, by measuring volume, pH, and titratable acidity, and calculating acid output. The hourly acid output is calculated and is referred to as the maximum acid output in poststimulation tests. Some laboratories consider calculation of the peak hourly acid output to be a more reproducible parameter. Peak acid output is determined by taking the total of the two highest 15-minute acid outputs and multiplying this figure by 2 to arrive at the hourly acid output.[1] When pentagastrin or histamine is administered, the peak acidity is usually seen within 15 to 45 minutes postinjection; whereas with Histalog, the peak appears between 45 and 75 minutes. An example of a complete gastric secretion analysis—including titratable acidity, acid output, maximum acid output, and peak acid output—is shown in Table 9–1. Normal values are again highly variable; however, normal individuals will usually not produce a maximum acid output over 40 mEq.[1] Persons who are unable to produce gastric acidity, as is seen in pernicious anemia and in some cases of gastric carcinoma, show no response to the stimulation, and the pH of the specimens does not fall below 6.0. Normal individuals will exhibit a fall in pH to below 3.5. Hourly basal and maximum acid outputs that are representative of conditions that produce abnormal gastric acidity are provided in Table 9–2.

TERMINOLOGY

Just as the theories concerning the significance and performance of the gastric analysis have changed, so has the terminology used to describe the variations in gastric acidity. The terms anacidity, achlorhydria, and hypochlorhydria have been used to describe the inability to produce gastric acid. However, because as their definitions were originally based on the distinction made between "free" and "combined" acid and the titration to pH 3.5, the use of three different terms has been abandoned. Only the term anacidity has been retained to designate the inability to produce gastric acid, and it is defined as failure to produce a pH less than 6.0 following gastric stimulation.[2]

SUMMARY

It appears that although the gastric analysis still holds a small role in the clinical laboratory, its value will probably continue to decline as more sophisticated procedures are developed and perfected.

REFERENCES

1. Baron, JH: Clinical Tests of Gastric Secretion: History, Methodology and Interpretation. Macmillan, London, 1978.
2. Cannon, DC: Examination of gastric and duodenal contents. In Henry, JB (ed): Clinical Diagnosis and Management by Laboratory Methods. WB Saunders, Philadelphia, 1984.
3. Freeman, JA and Beeler, MF: Laboratory Medicine: Urinalysis and Medical Microscopy. Lea & Febiger, Philadelphia, 1983.
4. Marks, IN, et al: The augmented histamine test: A review of 615 cases of gastroduodenal disease. S Afr J Surg 1:53–59, 1963.

STUDY QUESTIONS (Choose one best answer)

1. Gastric acidity is produced as the result of
    a. stimulation of the zymogen chief cells by gastrin to produce hydrochloric acid
    b. stimulation of the parietal cells by gastrin to produce hydrochloric acid
    c. stimulation of the parietal cells by signals from the vagus nerve
    d. stimulation of specialized G cells by pepsinogen to produce hydrochloric acid

2. The major constituents of gastric secretions are
    a. hydrochloric acid and mucus
    b. hydrochloric acid and bile
    c. hydrochloric acid and saliva
    d. hydrochloric acid and pepsin

3. Falsely decreased values for gastric acidity will occur if
    a. the patient is intubated while fasting
    b. the patient swallows large amounts of saliva
    c. the aspiration is performed continuously over the collection period
    d. the patient receives Histalog during the collection period

4. The recommended method of measuring gastric acidity is
    a. titrate with 0.1N NaOH to pH 3.5 with Töpfer's reagent, and report in degrees of acidity
    b. titrate with 0.1N NaOH to pH 3.5 with Töpfer's reagent, and report in milliequivalents per liter
    c. titrate with 0.1N NaOH to pH 7.0 with phenol red, and report in degrees of acidity
    d. titrate with 0.1N NaOH to pH 7.0 with phenol red, and report in milliequivalents per liter

5. At pH 7.0, phenol red changes from
    a. yellow to red
    b. red to yellow
    c. colorless to red
    d. red to colorless

6. Calculate the milliequivalents per liter of titratable acidity in a 15-ml specimen if 3.0 ml of 0.1N NaOH are used to titrate 10 ml to pH 7.0.

7. The above specimen represents the first 15-minute collection in a 1-hour basal specimen. Calculate the actual acid output of the specimen.

8. All 15-minute specimens of a 1-hour basal specimen produce results identical to those of the specimen in question 6. You would interpret this specimen to be

   a. indicative of Zollinger-Ellison syndrome
   b. indicative of pernicious anemia
   c. indicative of an improperly collected specimen
   d. indicative of normal gastric acidity

9. The preferred stimulant of gastric acidity for routine analysis is

   a. histamine
   b. Histalog
   c. pentagastrin
   d. insulin

10. Poststimulation specimens from persons with pernicious anemia will show

    a. no increased acidity and a pH above 6.0
    b. no increased acidity but a pH below 6.0
    c. increased acidity and a pH below 6.0
    d. increased acidity and a pH below 3.5

11. Poststimulation specimens for maximum acid output are

    a. collected, analyzed, and reported the same as basal specimens
    b. collected as a total 1-hour specimen, which is analyzed and reported as milliequivalents of acid output
    c. collected in the same manner as basal specimens but analyzed only for pH
    d. collected as a 1-hour specimen and analyzed for degrees of acidity

12. The inability to produce gastric acidity and a pH of less than 6.0 is termed

    a. achlorhydria
    b. hypochlorhydria
    c. anacidity
    d. hypoacidity

10

FECAL ANALYSIS

LEARNING OBJECTIVES

Upon completion of this chapter, the reader will be able to

1. describe the normal composition of feces
2. name a pathogenic and nonpathogenic cause, when presented with an abnormal description of fecal color
3. state the significance of increased neutrophils in a stool specimen
4. name the fecal fats stained by Sudan III and give the conditions under which they will stain
5. describe and interpret the microscopic results that will be seen when a specimen from a patient with steatorrhea is stained with Sudan III
6. state the principle of the chemical screening tests for "occult" blood
7. discuss the advantages and disadvantages of ortho-tolidine and guaiac as substrates in the "occult" blood screening test
8. briefly describe a chemical test performed on feces for each of the following: steatorrhea, fetal hemoglobin, pancreatic insufficiency, and carbohydrate intolerance

In the minds of most laboratory personnel, analysis of fecal specimens fits into the category of a "necessary evil." However, as an end product of body metabolism, feces do provide valuable diagnostic information. Routine fecal examination includes macroscopic, microscopic, and chemical analyses for the early detection of gastrointestinal bleeding, liver and biliary duct disorders, and malabsorption syndromes. Of equal diagnostic value is the detection and identification of pathogenic bacteria and parasites; however, these procedures are best covered in a microbiology textbook and will not be discussed here.

SPECIMEN COLLECTION

Collection of fecal specimens is seldom an easy task for the patient. Containers should be provided and patients instructed to collect the specimen in a clean container, such as a bedpan, and then to transfer the specimen to the laboratory container. They should be cautioned to avoid mixing the specimen with urine or contaminating it with water from the toilet that may contain chemical disinfectants. Specimens received in the laboratory vary from material collected on a physician's glove to 3-day specimens collected in paint cans. Small random specimens are adequate for performing qualitative tests for blood and microscopic examination for white blood cells and undigested materials, such as protein fibers and fecal fat. However, for quantitative analysis, timed specimens are needed in order to measure daily output. Due to the variability in bowel habits, the most representative timed sample is a 3-day collection.

PHYSIOLOGY

The normal fecal specimen contains bacteria, cellulose and other undigested foodstuffs, gastrointestinal secretions, bile pigments, cells from the intestinal walls, electrolytes, and water. Many species of bacteria make up the normal flora of the intestines and contribute to the digestive process. Bacterial metabolism produces the strong odor associated with feces. Disruption of the normal intestinal flora will lead to diarrhea, as will the introduction of pathogenic organisms. Digestive enzymes are secreted into the intestine primarily by the pancreas and function in the breakdown and absorption of proteins, carbohydrates, and fats. Major enzymes include trypsin, chymotrypsin, aminopeptidase, and lipase for the degradation of fats. Lack of one of these enzymes will cause an inability to digest and to absorb a particular foodstuff, resulting in the appearance of excess undigested material in the feces and the clinical symptoms of a malabsorption syndrome. Bile salts contribute to the digestion of fats; and bile pigment, in the form of urobilin, is believed to provide the normal brown color of the feces. Consequently, obstruction of the flow of bile into the intestine will lead to the production of light colored, fatty stools. Water and electrolytes are readily reabsorbed in the intestinal tract, and under normal conditions, the electrolyte concentration of the feces approximates that of the plasma. Should the intestinal contents become highly concentrated, excess water will remain in the intestine, and diarrhea will result. Constipation, on the other hand, provides time for additional water to be reabsorbed from the fecal material, producing small, hard stools.

The section of the laboratory to which routine fecal analysis is assigned varies among hospitals. Most commonly, the screening of random samples is included with the cultures and parasitology in the microbiology lab or is performed in urinalysis. Quantitative analyses are performed in the chemistry section.

FECES IN THE URINALYSIS LABORATORY

Routine fecal tests performed in the urinalysis laboratory include macroscopic observation of the color and consistency; microscopic examination for white blood cells, protein fibers, and fecal fat; and qualitative chemical tests for blood.

COLOR AND APPEARANCE

The first indication of gastrointestinal disturbances can often be provided by changes in the normal brown color of the feces. Of course, the appearance of abnormal fecal color may also be caused by the ingestion of highly pigmented foods and medications, so a differentiation must be made between this and a possible pathologic cause. Most frequently referred to is the black, tarry stool associated with upper gastrointestinal bleeding. Blood originating from the esophagus, stomach, or duodenum takes approximately 3 days to appear in the stool; during this time, degradation of hemoglobin produces the characteristic black color. Likewise, blood from the lower gastrointestinal tract requires less time to appear and will retain its original red color. Both black and red stools should be chemically tested for the presence of blood because ingestion of iron will often produce a black stool, and many foods and medications contain red pigment.

The appearance of pale stools can also cause concern; however, the recent administration of barium should first be considered, because this is a frequent nonpathogenic reason for grayish white stools. If barium has not been ingested, obstruction of the flow of bile pigment to the intestine and the lack of enzymes necessary for the digestion and absorption of fat must be investigated. In cases of fat malabsorption, termed steatorrhea,

TABLE 10–1. Macroscopic Stool Characteristics[2, 18]

APPEARANCE	POSSIBLE CAUSE
Black	Upper gastrointestinal bleeding Iron therapy Charcoal Bismuth (antacids)
Red	Lower gastrointestinal bleeding BSP dye Pyridium compounds Beets and food coloring Rifampin
Pale yellow, white, gray	Bile duct obstruction Barium
Yellow	Rhubarb
Green	Biliverdin Green vegetables Antibiotics
Bulky/frothy	Steatorrhea
Ribbonlike	Intestinal constriction
Mucus	Constipation Malignancy Colitis

the stools are often bulky and frothy and may appear pale or dark yellow. Stools from suspected cases of steatorrhea should be tested for the presence of excess fat.

Besides variations in color, additional abnormalities that may be observed during the macroscopic examination include the watery consistency present in diarrhea, and the small, hard stools seen with constipation. Slender, ribbonlike stools suggest an obstruction of the normal passage of material through the intestine. Also, the presence of mucus may indicate inflammation of the intestinal walls, and blood-streaked mucus shows excessive irritation of the walls. Observation of significant mucus or purulent exudate should be reported. A summary of the major macroscopic abnormalities is given in Table 10–1.

WHITE BLOOD CELLS

Microscopic examination of the feces for the presence of white blood cells is performed as a preliminary procedure in determining the cause of diarrhea. Neutrophils are seen in the feces in conditions that affect the intestinal wall, such as ulcerative colitis and infection with invasive bacterial pathogens. Organisms that cause diarrhea by toxin production, rather than intestinal wall invasion, do not cause the appearance of neutrophils in the feces. Therefore, the presence or absence of fecal neutrophils can provide the physician with diagnostic information prior to the isolation of a bacterial pathogen. As few as three neutrophils per high-power field can be indicative of an invasive condition.[2] Specimens may be examined as wet preparations stained with methylene blue, or they may be stained with Gram or Wright's stains.

QUALITATIVE FECAL FATS

Specimens from suspected cases of steatorrhea can be screened microscopically for the presence of excess fecal fat. Although this is a qualitative procedure that should be followed by a quantitative chemical measurement of fecal fat concentration, there is good correlation between the two procedures when the microscopic examination is carefully performed.[9] Lipids are found in the feces primarily in the form of neutral fats (triglycerides), fatty acid salts (soaps), and fatty acids. Their presence can be observed microscopically by staining with the dyes Sudan III, Sudan IV, or oil red O, of which Sudan III is the most routinely used. Neutral fats are readily stained by Sudan III and appear as large orange-red droplets often located near the edge of the coverslip.[10] Observation of more than 60 droplets per high-power field can be considered indicative of steatorrhea.

Soaps and fatty acids do not stain directly with Sudan III. Soaps must be converted to fatty acids by acetic acid, and fatty acids need to be melted to absorb the dye. Therefore, a second slide must be examined after the specimen has been mixed with acetic acid and heated. Examination of this slide will reveal stained droplets that represent not only the free fatty acids but also the fatty acids produced by hydrolysis of the soaps and the neutral fats (total fats). Normal specimens may contain as many as 100 small droplets, less than 4 microns in size, per high-power field.[4] Larger droplets, often more than 75 microns in size, are commonly seen in steatorrhea. Therefore, not only the number but also the size of the droplets must be considered when evaluating the slide for fatty acid content.[6] The presence of many large droplets may indicate the combination of several fatty acids, which would falsely decrease the droplet count.

Comparison of the results obtained from the initial examination representing neutral fat content and the posthydrolysis slide containing fatty acids can aid in determining whether steatorrhea is due to a lack of pancreatic enzymes or a malabsorption syndrome; an increase in neutral fat content indicates a deficiency in pancreatic enzymes. In contrast, steatorrhea caused by a malabsorption disorder would have a normal neutral fat content and increased total fats.[1]

The lipoidal absorption test provides an additional screening test for fecal fats and correlates well with quantitative fecal fat determinations. In normal persons an oral dose of iodinated poppyseed oil is readily absorbed from the intestine. The iodine is then split off and excreted by the kidneys. Urine is collected between 12 and 18 hours after ingestion and serially diluted to 1:32. Addition of starch to the serially diluted urine will detect the presence of iodine by producing a blue precipitate. In persons with steatorrhea who are unable to absorb the iodinated poppyseed oil, iodine will appear only in the 1:2 dilution; whereas normal persons will demonstrate iodine in dilutions ranging from 1:8 to 1:32.[5]

OCCULT BLOOD

By far the most frequently performed fecal analysis is the chemical screening test for the detection of "occult," or hidden, blood. As discussed earlier, bleeding in the upper gastrointestinal tract may produce a black, tarry stool, and bleeding in the lower gastrointestinal tract may result in an overtly bloody stool. However, because any bleeding in excess of 2 milliliters per 150 grams of stool is considered pathologically significant, and no visible signs of bleeding may be present with this amount of blood, chemical detection of the "occult" blood is necessary.[3] Originally used primarily to test suspected cases of gastrointestinal disease, the "occult" blood test has currently become widely used as a mass screening procedure for the early detection of colorectal cancer. The "occult" blood test will detect a high percentage of colorectal cancers while they are still in the localized stage. With proper physician follow-up, this has been shown to produce an 84 percent survival rate.[7]

Several different chemicals have been used to detect "occult" blood. All react in the same chemical manner but vary in their sensitivity. Listed in order of decreasing sensitivity, these compounds include benzidine, ortho-tolidine, and gum guaiac. Contrary to most chemical testing, the least sensitive reagent, guaiac, is preferred for routine testing. This choice can be better understood when one considers the chemical reaction taking place. This reaction utilizes the pseudoperoxidase activity of hemoglobin reacting with hydrogen peroxide to oxidize a colorless compound to a colored compound:

$$\text{Hemoglobin} \xrightarrow[\text{peroxidase}]{\text{pseudo-}} H_2O_2 \overset{O}{\rightarrow} \underset{\text{guaiac}}{\overset{\text{benzidine}}{\text{ortho-tolidine}}} \rightarrow \text{blue color}$$

Pseudoperoxidase activity, the key to this reaction, is also present in animal hemoglobin, certain vegetables, and some intestinal bacteria. Therefore, random samples collected from people under no dietary restrictions would produce false-positive reactions if tested with too sensitive a reagent. Benzidine, the most sensitive compound, is no longer available for clinical use because it possesses carcinogenic properties. Both ortho-tolidine and guaiac are available in commercial kits for laboratory use. Hematest (Ames Company, Elkhart, IN) supplies ortho-tolidine combined with tartaric acid, calcium acetate, and strontium peroxide in tablet form. When the tablet is placed on a fecal specimen and water is added, the tartaric acid and calcium acetate react with the strontium peroxide, releasing the peroxide to be acted upon by the hemoglobin pseudoperoxidases. If these peroxidases are present in the specimen, a blue color will be produced by the oxidized ortho-tolidine.[5] Because the sensitivity of ortho-tolidine may produce false-positive reactions, this test is most useful for monitoring patients with controlled dietary intake.

The products used in routine mass screening for ''occult'' blood include Hemoccult (Smith Kline Diagnostics, Sunnyvale, CA) and Fecatest (FinnPippette KY, Helsinki, Finland). Both kits contain guaiac-impregnated filter paper to which the fecal specimen and hydrogen peroxide are added. In the presence of hemoglobin pseudoperoxidase activity, a blue color will appear on the impregnated filter paper. Packaging of the guaiac-impregnated filter paper in individually sealed containers has facilitated the mass screening program for colorectal cancer by allowing persons at home to place a portion of the specimen on the paper and to mail it to the laboratory for testing. When possible, the fecal specimen placed on the filter paper should represent several portions of the stool, including the center, because intermittent bleeding may produce positive and negative areas in the same stool.[2] Hemoccult II containers have two windows for placement of stool from different areas. Persons collecting specimens at home must be cautioned to avoid contamination of the specimen with toilet bowl cleaners, which may interfere with the peroxidase reaction. Due to the decreased sensitivity of the guaiac reagent, it is recommended that at least three—ideally, six—different specimens be tested before a negative result is confirmed. False-negative results have also been reported from persons taking large doses of vitamin C, and false-positive reactions may occur in conjunction with iron therapy.[3] Additional methods for the detection of ''occult'' blood are currently under development and include an immunologic test that is specific for human hemoglobin and a chemical test that converts the heme portion of hemoglobin to porphyrin for analysis by fluorescence.[2]

FECES IN THE CHEMISTRY LABORATORY

QUANTITATIVE FECAL FATS

Quantitative chemical analysis of feces in the clinical laboratory is confined primarily to the measurement of fecal fat content for the confirmation of steatorrhea. As discussed earlier, quantitative fecal analysis requires the collection of at least a 3-day specimen. The patient must also maintain a regulated intake of fat prior to and during the collection period. Paint cans make excellent collection containers because the specimen must be homogenized prior to analysis, and this can be accomplished by placing the container on a conventional paint-can shaker. The method routinely used for fecal fat measurement is the Van de Kamer titration.[10] Fecal lipids are converted to fatty acids and titrated to a neutral end point with sodium hydroxide. The fat content is reported as grams of fat or fatty acids per 24 hours. Normal values are based on fat intake and range from 4 to 6 percent of the ingested fat.

APT TEST

Grossly bloody stools and vomitus are sometimes seen in neonates as the result of swallowing maternal blood during delivery. Should it be necessary to distinguish between the presence of fetal blood or that of maternal blood in an infant's stool or vomitus, the Apt test may be requested. The material to be tested is emulsified in water to release hemoglobin, and after centrifugation, 1 percent NaOH is added to the pink hemoglobin-containing supernatant. In the presence of alkali-resistant fetal hemoglobin, the solution will remain pink; whereas denaturation of the maternal hemoglobin will produce a yellow-brown supernatant.

TRYPSIN

Absence of the protein-digesting enzyme trypsin can be screened for by placing a small amount of stool emulsified in water on a piece of x-ray paper. In the presence of trypsin, the gelatin on the x-ray paper will be digested, leaving a clear area on the paper. Inability to digest the gelatin indicates a deficiency in trypsin production and is associated with pancreatic insufficiency. The gelatin test may be requested, in conjunction with more specific tests discussed in chapter 8, on infants suspected of having cystic fibrosis.

CARBOHYDRATES

Carbohydrate malabsorption or intolerance is primarily analyzed by serum tests; however, an increased concentration of carbohydrate can be detected by performing a copper reduction test on the fecal specimen. Carbohydrate testing is most valuable in assessing cases of infant diarrhea and may be accompanied by a pH determination, because utilization of the increased carbohydrate by intestinal bacteria will produce a lowered pH. The test is performed using a Clinitest tablet (Ames Company, Elkhart, IN) and 1 part stool emulsified in 2 parts water. As discussed in chapter 4, this is a general test for the presence of reducing substances, and a positive result would be followed by more specific serum carbohydrate tolerance tests, the most common of these being the D-xylose and lactose tolerance tests.

SUMMARY

A summary of fecal screening tests is presented in Table 10–2.

TABLE 10–2. Summary of Fecal Screening Tests

TEST	METHODOLOGY/PRINCIPLE	INTERPRETATION
Examination for neutrophils	Microscopic count of neutrophils in smear stained with methylene blue, Gram, or Wright's stain	3/hpf indicates condition affecting intestinal wall
Qualitative fecal fats	Microscopic examination of direct smear stain with Sudan III	60 large orange-red droplets indicate lack of pancreatic digestive enzymes
	Microscopic examination of smear heated with glacial acetic acid with Sudan III	100 small orange-red droplets or large droplets indicate malabsorption

TABLE 10–2. *Continued*

TEST	METHODOLOGY/PRINCIPLE	INTERPRETATION
Lipoidal absorption	Intestinal absorption of iodinated poppyseed oil produces urinary iodine detected by starch	Inability to demonstrate starch in a 1:8 dilution shows malabsorption
Occult blood	Pseudoperoxidase activity of hemoglobin liberates oxygen to oxidize gum guaiac	Blue color indicates gastrointestinal bleeding
Apt test	Addition of NaOH to hemoglobin-containing emulsion determines presence of maternal or fetal blood	Pink color indicates presence of fetal hemoglobin
Trypsin	Emulsified stool placed on x-ray paper to determine ability to digest gelatin	Inability to digest gelatin indicates lack of trypsin
Clinitest	Addition of emulsified stool to Clinitest to detect presence of reducing substances	Presence of reducing substances suggests carbohydrate malabsorption

REFERENCES

1. Anderson, DH: Celiac syndrome, determination of fat in feces; Reliability of two chemical methods and microscopic estimate: Excretion of feces and of fecal fat in normal children. Am J Dis Child 69(3):141–151, 1945.
2. Bradley, GM: Fecal analysis: Much more than an unpleasant necessity. Diagn Med 3(2):64–75, 1980.
3. Carroll, S: Fecal occult blood: Efficacy of testing measures. Nurse Pract 5(5):15–21, 1980.
4. Drummey, GD, Benson, JA, and Jones, CM: Microscopic examination of the stool for steatorrhea. N Engl J Med 264:85–87, 1961.
5. Freeman, JA and Beeler, MF: Laboratory Medicine: Urinalysis and Medical Microscopy. Lea & Febiger, Philadelphia, 1983.
6. Ghosh, SK, et al: Stool microscopy in screening for steatorrhea. J Clin Pathol 30:749–753, 1977.
7. Heim, C et al: Evaluation of positive hemoccult test results in a community screening program. J Tenn Med Assoc 79(12):755–758, 1986.
8. Kao, YS and Scheer, WD: Malabsorption, diarrhea, and examination of feces. In Henry, JB (ed): Clinical Diagnosis and Management by Laboratory Methods. WB Saunders, Philadelphia, 1979.
9. Semko, V: Fecal fat microscopy. Am J Gastroenterol 75(3):204–208, 1981.
10. Van de Kamer, JH, et al: A rapid method for determination of fat in feces. J Biol Chem 177:347–355, 1949.

STUDY QUESTIONS (Choose one best answer)

1. The normal brown color of the feces is produced by
   a. undigested foodstuffs
   b. urobilin
   c. pancreatic enzyme
   d. cellulose

2. Diarrhea can result from all of the following except
   a. disruption of the normal intestinal bacterial flora
   b. addition of pathogenic organisms to the normal intestinal flora
   c. increased reabsorption of intestinal water and electrolytes
   d. increased concentration of fecal electrolytes

3. Stools from persons with steatorrhea will contain excess amounts of
   a. barium sulfate
   b. mucus
   c. blood
   d. fat

4. Which of the following pairings of stool appearance and cause does not match?
   a. black, tarry = blood
   b. yellow-green = barium sulfate
   c. pale, frothy = steatorrhea
   d. yellow-white = bile duct obstruction

5. Microscopic examination of stools provides preliminary information as to the cause of diarrhea because
   a. neutrophils will be present in conditions caused by toxin-producing bacteria
   b. neutrophils will be present in conditions that affect the intestinal wall
   c. red and white blood cells will be present if the cause is bacterial
   d. neutrophils will be present if the condition is of nonbacterial etiology

6. Large orange-red droplets seen on direct microscopic examination of stools mixed with Sudan III represent
   a. fatty acids
   b. soaps
   c. neutral fats
   d. cholesterol

7. Microscopic examination of stools mixed with Sudan III and glacial acetic acid and then heated will show small orange-red droplets that represent
   a. soaps
   b. fatty acids and soaps
   c. fatty acids and neutral fats
   d. fatty acids, soaps, and neutral fats

8. Examination of direct and posthydrolysis slides for fat droplets reveals a normal neutral fat content and an increased amount of fatty acids. This is indicative of
   a. steatorrhea due to increased triglyceride consumption
   b. steatorrhea due to lack of pancreatic enzymes
   c. steatorrhea due to inability to convert fatty acids to soaps
   d. steatorrhea due to a malabsorption disorder

9. The term "occult" blood describes blood that
   a. is produced in the lower gastrointestinal tract
   b. is produced in the upper gastrointestinal tract
   c. is not visibly apparent in the stool specimen
   d. produces a black, tarry stool

10. Tests for the detection of "occult" blood rely on the

    a. reaction of hemoglobin with hydrogen peroxide
    b. pseudoperoxidase activity of hemoglobin
    c. reaction of hemoglobin with ortho-tolidine
    d. pseudoperoxidase activity of hydrogen peroxide

11. Gum guaiac is preferred over ortho-tolidine for "occult" blood in mass screening tests because

    a. there is less interference from dietary hemoglobin
    b. ortho-tolidine is less sensitive
    c. gum guaiac reacts equally with formed and watery stools
    d. filter paper is more easily impregnated with gum guaiac

12. In the Van de Kamer method for quantitative fecal fat determinations,

    a. fecal lipids are homogenized and titrated to a neutral end point with sodium hydroxide
    b. fecal lipids are measured gravimetrically after ashing
    c. fecal lipids are converted to fatty acids prior to titrating with sodium hydroxide
    d. fecal lipids are measured by spectrophotometer after addition of Sudan III

ANSWER KEY

CHAPTER 1

1. c	7. b	13.	Glycolysis had occurred; dilute random specimen		
2. a	8. d				
3. b	9. b	14.	2-hour postprandial with fasting specimen		
4. d	10. c				
5. d	11. d				
6. b	12. b				

CHAPTER 2

1. d	9. d	17. d	25. b
2. d	10. c	18. c	26. c
3. c	11. d	19. b	27. b
4. d	12. a	20. c	28. a
5. b	13. c	21. d	29. d
6. a	14. d	22. b	30. 675 ml/min
7. b	15. 100 ml/min	23. b	31. c
8. d	16. 100 ml/min	24. c	32. e, c, f, a, b

CHAPTER 3

1. c	5. d	9. a	13. b	17. d
2. a	6. b	10. d	14. c	18. b
3. b	7. a	11. 1.009	15. d	
4. c	8. c	12. c	16. a	

CHAPTER 4

1. b	10. a	19. d	28. b
2. c	11. d	20. c	29. c
3. c	12. d	21. a	30. a
4. d	13. c	22. b	31. b
5. b	14. a	23. c	32. d
6. a	15. c	24. b	33. c
7. d	16. b	25. d	34. c, e, f, c, c, d,
8. c	17. b	26. c	g, b, f, b
9. d	18. c	27. d	

35. a. yes
b. no
c. yes
d. no

36. a. The patient's clinical symptoms suggest a urinary tract infection. Large doses of ascorbic acid may be interfering with the nitrite and leukocyte tests.
    b. Red blood cell protein would contribute to the urinary protein, as would leukocytes.
    c. Amber urine suggesting a concentrated specimen is also produced by large doses of vitamin A (carotene).
    d. Bacterial breakdown of urine urea to ammonia and vegetarian diets raise urinary pH.

CHAPTER 5

1. c	6. a	11. b	16. c
2. b	7. b	12. d	17. d
3. a	8. c	13. d	18. a
4. c	9. c	14. b	19. d
5. d	10. b	15. b	20. a

21. a. triple phosphate
    b. ammonium biurate
    c. calcium oxalate
    d. calcium carbonate

22. d, a, e, b   24. d

23. b   25. a

26. a. positive blood and cloudy specimen
    b. positive nitrite suggests urinary infection
    c. protein may be found with casts or may be due only to RBCs, WBCs, and bacteria
    d. positive nitrite caused by bacterial reduction of urinary nitrate

27. a. positive blood; however, RBCs may have lysed in dilute alkaline urine
    b. positive nitrite and clinical symptoms suggest urinary infection
    c. high pH favors formation of triple phosphate crystals
    d. positive nitrite caused by bacterial reduction of urinary nitrate

28. Concentrated urine containing casts and RBCs is frequently seen after strenuous exercise. After a period of rest, the results should return to normal.

29. a. Did you recheck the pH and verify crystal identification?
    b. Did you call the result to the physician?
    c. Did the patient have a recent IVP?
    d. Did you confirm reactivity of dipstick, and did you consider yeast or oil droplets?

30. Inspect control and check lot number. Retest. Use new control. Use new reagent strips. Test new lot number. Notify supervisor.

CHAPTER 6

1. c	7. d	13. c	19. a
2. c	8. a	14. d	20. b
3. d	9. d	15. b	21. d
4. a	10. a	16. b, a, a, b, b	22. b
5. b	11. d	17. c	23. c
6. c	12. d	18. c	

CASE STUDIES

1. A diet high in fresh Hawaiian pineapple would produce a false-positive 5-HIAA. The result would return to normal after dietary restriction.
2. The blue color in the catheter bag could be caused by the oxidation of urinary indican to indigo blue. Bobby's symptoms are consistent with Hartnup disease, which can be controlled by dietary regulation. Amino acid chromatography should be performed on the urine to check for a generalized aminoaciduria.
3. The ferric chloride tube test and the DNPH test are consistent with phenylketonuria and maple syrup urine disease. False-negative PKU results on first specimens are most frequently seen in female infants; therefore, this test should be repeated, and urinary amino acid chromatography should be performed.

CHAPTER 7

1. b	9. c	17. a	25. b
2. c	10. d	18. d	26. d
3. c	11. b	19. b	27. d
4. a, a, b, b	12. a	20. c	28. b
5. c	13. c	21. a	29. b
6. 150/μl	14. b	22. c	30. a
7. a	15. a	23. d	
8. 3000/μl	16. d	24. d	

CASE STUDIES

1. Results suggest a bacterial meningitis. Other tests could include a CSF lactate and a Limulus lysate test for the presence of gram-negative organisms. There is at least a 10 percent possibility of a false-negative Gram stain and culture. Blood cultures could be helpful.
2. Clinical symptoms and initial test results suggest multiple sclerosis, which can be confirmed with protein electrophoresis and an IgG index.
3. Viral = lactate, LD isoenzymes
   Tubercular = acid-fast stain, lactate, glucose
   Fungal = Gram stain, India ink, lactate, glucose

CHAPTER 8

1. c	10. c	19. b	28. a
2. c	11. b	20. c	29. d
3. a	12. d	21. c	30. c
4. c	13. b	22. b	31. b
5. d	14. d	23. a	32. c
6. d	15. c	24. d	33. c
7. c	16. c	25. b	34. c
8. d	17. a	26. c	35. b
9. c	18. b	27. b	36. b

CHAPTER 9

1. b	4. d	7. 0.45 mEq acid	10. a
2. d	5. a	8. d	11. a
3. b	6. 30 mEq/liter	9. c	12. c

CHAPTER 10

1. b	4. b	7. d	10. b
2. c	5. b	8. d	11. a
3. d	6. c	9. c	12. c

INDEX

An "f" following a page number indicates a figure. A "t" following a page number indicates a table.

Abnormal crystals, 99–102
    major characteristics of, 101t
ABO blood grouping, 166
Acetest, 68
Acetic, 68
Acetic acid, 169, 202
Acetoacetic acid, 67
Acetone, 67
Acetylacetone, 127
Acetylcholinesterase activity, 183
Achlorhydria, 196
Acid base content, 60. *See also* pH
Acid output, determination of gastric, 196
Acid phosphatase, test for, 166
Acid urine, crystals in, 99
Acid-albumin turbidity test, 128
Acidosis, pH and, 60
Active transport, 17–18
Acute glomerulonephritis, 32–33
Addis, Thomas, 2, 88
Addis count, elements in, 88
ADH. *See* Antidiuretic hormone
Aerobes/anaerobes, Gram stain test for, 179
Agarose gel, 148
Albinism, 122
Albumin, 61
    CSF specimens, 143–144
    major CSF protein, 146
    tubular disorders, 62
Albuminuria. *See* Proteinuria
Aldosterone, 17, 19
"Alkali lover," 122
Alkaline biuret-protein chelate formation, 147
Alkaline phosphatase determination, 179
Alkaline urine, 99
Alkalosis, pH and, 60
Alkaptonuria, 119, 122
Alpha fetal protein levels, 183
Alpha globulins, 147
α-keto-β-methylvaleric, 123
α-ketoglutarate, 149

α-ketoisocaproic, 123
α-ketoisovaleric, 123
Alveolar stability, 181–182
American Diabetes Association, 65
Ames-N-Multistix, 60. *See also* Multistix
Amino acid chromatography, 123
Amino acid disorders, 119–123
Amino acids, 125
Aminoaciduria, 121, 126
Aminolevulinic acid (ALA), 126
Aminostat-FLM test, 182–183
Ammonia, urinary, titratable acidity and, 32
Ammonium biurate crystals, 99
Ammonium concentration: calculation of, 32
Amniocentesis procedure, 180
Amniotic fluid, 180–183, 183t
Amoeboid migration, 93
Amorphous phosphates, 45, 99
Ampicillin crystals, 99, 102
Amylase test, 177, 179
Amyloid material, 62
Anacidity, defined, 196
Anencephaly, 183
Antidiuretic hormone (ADH), 10
    concentration of in plasma and urine, measurement of, 29
    function of, 19
    specific gravity measure and, 46
Anti-intrinsic factor, test for, 192
Antiparietal cell antibodies, test for, 192
Anuria, 3, 9
Apatite crystals, 169
APT test, 204
Argentaffin cells, 125
Arginine, as amino acid, 125
Arteriole
    afferent, 14, 15f, 17
    efferent, 14–15, 15f
Arthritis
    origin of, 173

synovial fluid and, 168
synovial fluid lactate levels and, 171
Arthrocentesis, 167
Artifacts, in urine, 102
Ascites, defined, 177
Ascitic fluid, 177–179
    chemical examination of, 179
Asparagus, urine odor and, 50
Aspartamine, 119
Astra, 147
Automated Chemistry Analyzer, 147
Azotemia, 9
Azure A dye, 128

Bacillus subtilis, 121
Bacteria, 5, 97–102
    gram-negative, 76
    non-nitrate-reducing gram-positive, 76
    turbidity and, 45
Bacterial meningitis, 146, 148, 149
Bacterial metabolism, in feces, 200
Bacterial peritonitis, 179
Bacteriuria, 76
Barium, 200
Basal lamina, 16, 16f
Beer's law, 147
Beets, red urine and, 43
Bence-Jones protein, 10
    multiple myeloma and, 62
    unique solubility of, 63–64
Benedict's solution, 66
Benedict's test, 122
Benzidine, 202, 203
Beta globulins, 147
β₂ microglobulin, glomerular filtration test and, 23
Bile, 179
Bile pigment, 200
Bile salts, 200
Bilirubin, 5, 70–73
    in amniotic fluid, 181

Bilirubin—*Continued*
  clinical significance of, 71–72
  errors in testing, 73
  hepatitis virus and, 43
  importance of test for, 70
  oxidation tests for, 72
  presence of, 43
  production of, 71
  summary of clinical significance of urinary, 72
Bilirubin crystals, 102
Bilirubin diglucuronide, 71
Bilirubinuria, 71
Biliverdin, 72
Birefringence, defined, 169
Birth defects, amniotic fluid analysis and, 180–183
Biuret method, CSF analysis and, 147
BJP (Bence Jones protein), 10
Black stools, 200
Bleeding, in gastrointestinal tract, 202
Blood
  occult, 202–203
  in pleural fluid, 176
  in stool, 200–201
  uneven distribution of, 140
  in urine
    color variations in, 43
    significance of, 68–70
    summary of clinical significance of, 69
Blood glucose test, 148
Blood pressure, glomerular, 17
Blood urea nitrogen (BUN), elevation of, 32–33
Blood-brain barrier, 138
"Blue diaper syndrome," 124
Body fluids, miscellaneous, 160–184
Body size
  calculation of, 25
  nomogram for determination of, 26f
  renal function/blood flow and, 15–16
Bowman's capsule, 15f, 16
Bright, Richard, 2
Broad casts, 97
Bromthymol blue, 61
BUN (blood urea nitrogen), 10
Butanol, use of in testing, 74

Calcium acetate, 203
Calcium oxalate crystals, 99
Calcium phosphate, 99
Calcium pyrosphosphate crystals, 169
CAP. *See* College of American Pathologists
Capillaries, fenestrated, 17
Capillary tuft, 16
Carbohydrate tolerance tests, 204

Carbohydrates, screening test for malabsorption or intolerance of, 204
Carbonates, cloudiness and, 45
Carcinoembryonic antigen (CEA), 177, 179
Casts, 94–97
  microscopic examination of, 89
  types of, 95t
Catheter, 9
Cation exchange dipsticks, 127
CEA (carcinoembryonic antigen) levels, 179
Cell count, CSF specimens, 141
Centrifugation
  CSF specimen, 143
  in microscopic analysis, 89
Cerebrospinal fluid (CSF), 137–153
  analysis, 152
  appearance of, 139
    clinical significance of, 140t
  chemical composition of, 138
  in chemistry laboratory, 146–150
  collection of, 138–139
  flow of, 138f
  function of, 137–138
  in hematology laboratory, 139–146
  in microbiology laboratory, 150–152
  predominant cells in, 145t
  in serology laboratory,152
  serum protein correlations, 146t
  specimen collection tubes, 139f
  summary of chemistry tests of, 150
  terms used for, 139
Cerebrospinal fluid chemicals
  as clinically important, 146–150
  normal/plasma values, 146
Cerebrospinal fluid glucose, 148–149
  evaluation of, 148
Cerebrospinal fluid glutamine, 149
Cerebrospinal fluid lactate, meningitis and, 149
Cerebrospinal fluid protein
  fractionation of, 148
  measuring, 147
Cerebrospinal lactic dehydrogenase, 149–150
Ceruloplasmin, 147
Cetyltrimethylammonium bromide (CTAB) turbidity test, 128
Chemstrip, 55
  comparison of with Multistix, 56–57
  urobilinogen, 74
Chloride, 184
Chloroform, 75
Chocolate agar, 173
Cholesterol crystals, 99, 102, 169
Choroid plexus cells, 144–145
Christians, Dr. Henry, 88
Chromatography, thin-layer, 67, 182
Chromogens, 23

oxidized, 69–70
Chylous material
  identifying, 176
  in peritoneal fluid, 179
Cirrhosis, 179
  bilirubinuria and, 71
Clearance substance, calculation of, 23–25
Clearance tests, 22–23
Clinilab, 49, 59
Clini-Tek, 59, 60
Clinitest
  appraisal of, 66
  homogentisic acid, 122
  infant diarrhea and, 204
Clorets, 43
Clot formation, traumatic tap and, 140–141
Cloudiness, causes of, 45
"Coffin lids," 99
College of American Pathologists (CAP), 103
  quality control program of, 107
Colligative property, 28
Colloidal gold test, 148
Color
  changes in, 5
  urinary, 42–45
    abnormal, 43–45
    brown/black, 43
    clinical significance of, 43
    as diagnostic tool, 42
    laboratory correlation of, 44–45t
    medication and, 43–44
    normal, 42–43
    red, 43
    urine concentration and, 43
Color reactions, interpretation of, 55
Colorectal cancer, detection of, 202
Colorimetric end-point reaction, 147
Coma, CSF glutamine test and, 149
"Combined" (organic) acid, 193
Condoms, specimen collection and, 162
Constipation, 200
Convoluted tubules, 15f
  distal, 15
  proximal, 15
Coomassie brilliant blue G-250 dye, 147
Copper reduction test, 66. *See also* Benedict's test; Clinitest
  comparison of with glucose oxidase, 66–67
  in newborn screening programs, 129
Cortex, of kidney, 15, 15f
Corticosteroid crystals, 169
Cotugno, Domenico, 137
Countercurrent mechanisms, 18
Counterimmunoelectrophoresis (CIE), 152
Count-10 System, 88
Cranberry juice, 61

Creatinine, 2
  urine concentration and, 117
Creatinine clearance test
  clinical significance of, 25
  disadvantages of, 23
  glomerular filtration rate and, 23
  value of, 25
Cryptococcus neoformans, 151
Crystalluria, renal calculi and, 102
Crystals
  synovial fluid, 169, 171t
  urinary, 98–102
    formation of, 60, 98
    identification of, 98
    normal/abnormal, 100t, 101t
Cyanide-nitroprusside test
  cystinuria and, 125
  homocystinuria and, 126
Cylindroids, 94
Cylindroiduria, 94
Cystic fibrosis
  defined, 183–184
  diagnosis of, 183
  indicators of, 184
Cystine, as amino acid, 125
Cystine crystals, 99, 102
Cystine metabolism, disorders of,
    125–126
Cystinosis, 126
Cystinuria, 102, 125
Cystitis, 36, 75
Cystoscope, 9
Cytocentrifugation, 90, 143
  recovery chart, 144t
"Cytodiagnostic urinalysis," 90
Cytogenic analysis, 180
Cytologic examination
  gastric contents, 192
  pericardial fluid, 177
  peritoneal fluid, 179

"Degrees of acidity," 193
Dekker, Frederik, 2
Dermatan sulfate, 128
Dewpoint
  defined, 29
  measurement of, 28, 29
Dextran, 50
Diabetes insipidus, 77
  causes of, 4
  diagnosis of, 29
  polyuria and, 3
Diabetes mellitus, 3
  glucose test and, 64
  nephropathy and, 62
  polyuria and, 3
  yeast cells and, 98
Diarrhea
  causes of, 200, 201
  infant, test for, 204
Diazo reaction, 72
Differential count, 143–146
  abnormal cells, 144–145
  normal cells, 144

Digital Urinometer, 49
Dipstick, specific gravity and, 49
Diuresis, 9
DNA analysis, 166
D-xylose tolerance test, 204
Dye binding ability, 147
Dysuria, 9

Edema, 9
Edwin Smith Surgical Papyrus, 1
Ehrlich reaction, porphyrinuria and,
    126
Ehrlich-reactive compounds, 73
  interference by, 74
Ehrlich's reagent, 73
Ehrlich's tube test, 73–74
  reactions to, 75f
Ehrlich units, 74
Electrophoresis, 148
Elevated protein, clinical signifi-
    cance of, 147
-emia, 9
Endogenous procedure, defined, 23
Endoscopy, 192
Endothelial cells, 17
Enzyme function, disruption of, 118
Enzyme-linked immunosorbent assay
    method (Elisa), 152
Eosin-nigrosin stain, 165
Eosinophils, 145
Ependymal cells, 144–145
Epithelial cell casts, 96–97
Epithelial cells
  renal tubular, 93, 94
  squamous, 45, 94
  transitional (caudate), 94
  turbidity and, 45
  types of, 94
Equipment, in urinalysis laboratory,
    107–108
Errors, results of correction of, 104t
Erythrocytic malfunctions, 126
Escherichia coli, 152
Escherichia coli peroxidase, 70
Esterases, 77
Ethylenediaminetetraacetic acid
    (EDTA) (sequestrin) tube, 167
Exogenous procedure, 23
External quality control programs,
    107
Exudates
  classification of, 175t
  defined, 174
  laboratory differentiation of
    transudates and, 175t

Facilities, in urinalysis laboratory,
    109–110
Falling drop method, 49
Fanconi syndrome, 126
Fat malabsorption, 200–201
Fat metabolism
  clinical reasons for increase in, 67

products of, 67
Fatty acid salts (soaps), testing of,
    202
Fatty acids, testing of, 202
Fatty casts, 97
Fecal analysis, 199–205
Fecal fats
  measurement for concentration of,
    202
  qualitative, 202
  quantitative, 203–204
Fecal screening tests, summary of,
    204–205t
Fecal specimens
  collection of, 199–200
  physiology of, 200
Fecatest, 203
Feces
  appearance of, 200–201
  in chemistry laboratory, 203–204
  diagnostic value of, 199
  significance of color of, 200–201
  in urinalysis laboratory, 200–203
Ferric chloride test
  DNPH and, 123
  homogentisic acid, 122
  melanin and, 122
  Phenistix test and, 121
Fertility, sperm count as measure of,
    163
Fetal age, determination of, 183
Fetal anemia, 180–181
Fetal distress, 181
Fetal lung maturity (FLM), measure-
    ments for, 182–183
Fetal maturity, 181–183
Fetus, in amniotic sac, 180f
Filtered bicarbonate
  reabsorption of, 20f
  tubular secretion and, 19
Filtered phosphate, reaction of se-
    creted hydrogen ion with, 21f
Filtrate (ultrafiltrate of plasma), anal-
    ysis of, 17
Filtration process, factors affecting,
    16, 16f
First-order red compensator,
    169–170
Fishberg test, 26–27
Fisherbrand, 88
5-Hydroxyindoleacetic acid
    (5-HIAA), 124, 125
Fluorescent screening, 127–128
Fluorescent treponemal antibody ab-
    sorption (FTA-ABS) test, 152
Fluoroscopic examination, 193
Foam Stability Index, 183
Foam test, 72
  fetal lung maturity, 183
Focal glomerulonephritis, 36
Folling, Ivan, 119
Formed elements, presence of as in-
    dicative of disease, 2
Fouchet's reagent, 72
"Free" (hydrochloric) acid, 193

Free water clearance, calculation of, 29–30
Freezing point depression, measurement of, 28
Fructosuria, test for, 129
Fungal meningitis, 146
    India ink preparation and, 151
    symptoms of, 149

Galactose, 67
Galactosemia, 121
Galactosuria, 67
    testing for, 129
Gastric acidity
    basal, diagnostic value of, 194
    formation of, 192–193
    measurement of, 192–194
    poststimulation, 194–196
Gastric analysis, 192–196
    normal/abnormal results, 196t
    sample, 195t
Gastric carcinoma, 196
Gastric secretions
    collection of, 193
    contents of, 193
    titration procedures for, 193–194
Gastrin, 193
Genitalia, diagram of male, 161f
Gerhardt's test, 68
Ghost cells, 93
Gibson and Cooke, technique of, 184
"Glitter cells," 93
Glomerular bleeding, blood color and, 43
Glomerular filtration, 16–17, 16f
Glomerular filtration tests, 22–25
Glomerular membrane, damage to, 62
Glomerulonephritis
    acute, 32–33
    chronic, 33
    crescentic, 32
    focal, 36
    membranous, 33
    mesangiocapillary, 33–36
    streptococcal, 62
Glomerulus, 16
Glucose, 4, 64–67
    specific gravity of, 48
    urinary, summary of clinical significance of, 65
Glucose oxidase procedure, 65
    comparison of with Clinitest, 66–67
Glucose test
    peritoneal fluid, 179
    pleural fluid, 177, 179
    synovial fluid, 172
Glucose tolerance test (GTT), 64–65
Glucosuria. See Glycosuria
Glutamine test, 149
Glycolysis, 148
Glycosaminoglycans. See Mucopolysaccharides

Glycosuria (glucosuria), 9, 18, 64–65
Gout, uric acid crystals and, 99
Gradients, defined, 17
Gram stain, 150–151
    aerobes/anaerobes, 179
    feces, 201
    synovial fluid, 172–173
Granular casts, 97
Granulocyte count, 179
Greiss reaction, 75
Group B streptococci, 152
GTT (glucose tolerance test), 10
GU (genitourinary), 10
Guaiac, 202–203
Gum guaiac. See Guaiac
Guthrie's test, 120–121f

Haptoglobin content, 69, 147
Harrison spot test, 72
Hartnup disease, 124
Hart's test, 68
HCG (human chorionic gonadotropin), 10
Hematest, 203
Hematocrit, 176
Hematoidin crystals, 144
Hematuria, 9, 68–69
    renal calculi and, 92
    symptoms of, 68
    tests for, 69, 70
Heme formation
    pathway of, 127f
    porphyrin metabolism and, 126–128
Hemoccult, 203
Hemocytometer, 142
    Addis count and, 88
Hemoglobin
    free, 68, 69
    pseudoperoxidase activity of, 69
    in red urine, 43
Hemoglobin degradation, 71f
Hemoglobinuria, 68–69
    plasma and, 43
    symptoms of, 68
    tests for, 69, 70
Hemolysis, intravascular, 69
Hemolytic disease of newborns, 180
Hemophilus, 173
Hemophilus influenzae, 152
Hemorrhage, elevated CSF protein and, 147
Hemorrhagic trauma, 179
Hemosiderin, 99
Hemosiderin granules, 144
Hemothorax, 176
Heparan sulfate, 128
Heparinized tube, 167
Hepatic malfunction, 126
Hepatitis
    bilirubin and, 43
    bilirubinuria and, 71
Hippocrates, on uroscopy, 1–2
Hippurate, radioactive, use of to

measure renal blood flow, 31
Histalog, 194–196
Histamine, 194–196
Histidinemia, 121
Histiocytes, 94
HLA testing, 166
HLA-B$_{12}$ antigen, 36
Hoeltge and Ersts on control of sediment constituents, 105–107
Hoesch test, 127
Homocystinuria, 121, 126
Homogentisic acid, 122
    tests for, 43, 122
Homogentisic acid oxidase, 122
hpf (high power field), 10
Hunter's syndrome, 128
Hurler's syndrome, 128
Hyaline casts, 96
Hyaluronate, 168
Hydration, urine concentration and, 25
Hydrochloric acid
    function of, 192–193
Hydrogen ion
    collection and measurement of, 193
    excretion of excess, 19
    function of secretion of, 19
    secreted
        reaction of with ammonia, 21f
        reaction of with filtered phosphate, 21f
Hydrogen peroxide, in testing, 69–70
Hydrometer, 10. See also Urinometer
Hydrostatic pressure: filtration and, 17
Hypersthenuria, 9
Hypersthenuric, 50
Hypochlorhydria, 196
Hyposthenuria, 9
Hyposthenuric, 50

Ictotest, 72
IgA in CSF, 147
IgG in CSF, 147
IgG index, formula for, 148
IgG profile, 148
Immunofluorescent antibody-coated bacteria (ACB) test, 36
Immunologic agglutination test, 182
Inborn errors of metabolism
    alkaptonuria as, 122
    cystinosis as, 126
    disruption of enzyme function as, 118
    galactosuria as, 67
    maple syrup urine disease and, 123
    pentosuria as, 129
    porphyrias as, 126
India ink preparation, fungal meningitis and, 151
Indican, 124

Infants. *See also* Newborns
xanthochromia in, 140
In-house controls, 105, 106–107t
Instrumentation, in urinalysis laboratory, 107
Insulin hypoglycemia test, 196
Intubation, 193
Inulin, glomerular filtration testing and, 23
Iodinated poppy seed oil, 202
Isoleucine, as amino acid, 123
Isothenuria, 9
Isothenuric, defined, 49
IVP (intravenous pyelogram), 10

Jaundice
clinical, 71
urine bilirubin and urobilinogen in, 72t
Joint Commission of Accreditation of Hospitals (JCAH), 103
Joint disorders
classification and pathologic significance of, 167t
summary of laboratory findings in, 168t
"Joint fluid," 166
Juvenile diabetes, ketonuria and, 67

Keratan sulfate, 128
Keto acids, maple syrup urine disease and, 123
Ketones, 4, 67–68
diabetic, 50
glucose oxidase tests and, 65
urinary, summary of clinical significance of, 67
Ketonuria, 9, 67
Ketosis, 68
KOVA, 88

Lactic acid, influence of, 29
Lactic dehydrogenase
separation of, 150
test, 174
Lactose, appearance of, 67
Lactose tolerance test, 204
Latex agglutination method, 152
Lavage fluids, analysis of, 177
LD isoenzymes, value of, 150
LE cells, 169
Lead poisoning
porphyrinuria and, 126
test for, 127
Lecithin
function of, 181
measurement of, 182
Lecithin-sphingomyelin (L/S) ratio, 181
Leucine, as amino acid, 123
Leucine crystals, 99, 102, 121
Leukemia, uric acid crystals and, 99
Leukocyte (WBC) count, CSF specimens and, 141

Leukocyte decarboxylase test, 123
Leukocyte esterase reagent strip test, 162, 181
Leukocytes, 77
chemical test for, 46
reagent strip reaction, 77
renal tubular epithelial cells and, 93
summary of clinical significance of, 77
Levodopa, 68
Light reflection, principle of, 59
Limulus lysate test, 151–152
Lipemic serum, influence of, 29
Lipids, in feces, 202
Lipid-storage diseases, epithelial cells and, 94
Lipoidal absorption test, 202
Liver disease
early diagnosis of, 73
tyrosyluria and, 121
Loop of Henle, 15, 15f, 18
Low power field (lpf), 10, 89
lpf (low power field), 10, 89
Lumadex-FSI, 183
Lung surface lipids, 182
measurement of, 183
Lupus erythematosus, 62, 173
Lymphocytes, monocytes and, 144
Lysine, as amino acid, 125

Macrophages, CSF specimens, 144
Malabsorption syndrome, clinical symptoms of, 200
Maple syrup urine disease, 50, 121, 123
Medulla, of kidney, 15, 15f
osmotic gradient in, 19
Melanin
deficiency of, 122
testing for, 43
Melanogen, 122
Melanoma, malignant, 122
Melanuria, 119, 122
Melituria, as symptom, 129
Membranoproliferative glomerulonephritis, 33–36
Membranous glomerulonephritis, 33
Meningitis
defined, 144
diagnosis of, 146
differential diagnosis of, 151t
elevated CSF protein and, 147
LD isoenzymes and, 150
microbiology laboratory and, 150, 151t
symptoms of, 144
types of, 146
Menstrual contamination, 92
Mesangiocapillary glomerulonephritis, 33–36
Mesothelial cells, pleural, 177
Metabolic acidosis, 19
Metabolic constituents/conditions, in routine urinalysis, 117t

Metabolic disease, system of screening for, 118f
Metabolites, abnormal urinary, according to functional defect, 118, 119t
Metastatic carcinoma cells, 146
Methyl red, 61
Methylene blue stain, 201
Microalbumin, 62
Microprotein Rapid Stat Kit, 147
Microscopy
bright-field, 89, 90
interference-contrast, 90
Milliosmole (mOsm), 28
Millon test, 122
Minimal change disease, 36
Molality, 28
Molarity, 28
Monoclonal immunoglobulin light chains. *See* Bence-Jones protein
Monocytes, lymphocytes and, 144
Mononuclear cells, 169
Monosodium urate crystals, 169
Mosenthal test, 27
Motility, of sperm, 163–164
Mousy odor, 119
MPS papers, 128
Mucin clot test, 168, 169
Mucopolysaccharide disorders, 128
Mucus, 98
Multiple myeloma, Bence-Jones protein and, 62, 64
Multiple sclerosis
banding in, 148
IgG and, 148
symptoms of, 144, 145
Multiple test strips, ketone tests and, 67
Multistix, 55
comparison of with Chemstrip, 56–57
Multistix leukocyte esterase test, 143
Myoglobin, 43, 70
Myoglobinuria, plasma and, 43, 69, 70

NaCl, osmometer's use of, 29
Needle aspirations, procedures for, 173
Neisseria, 173
Neisseria meningitidis, 152
Nephelometry, 46, 63, 148
Nephritis, 9
Nephrology, 9
Nephron
composite view of, 13–14, 15f
movement of substances in, 20f
relation of parts of to lab tests, 21, 22f
relationship of to kidney, 13, 14f
Nephropathy, diabetic, 62
Nephrotic syndrome, 33
Neubauer counting chamber
CSF specimens, 142f

Neubauer counting chamber—
    Continued
    red/white blood cell counts, 164f
    serous fluids, 176
    sperm count and, 163
    synovial fluid, 168–169
Neubauer formula, 143
Neural tube disorders, 183
Neurosyphilis, 152
Neutral fats (triglycerides), test for,
    202
Neutrophils
    in feces, 201
    in synovial fluid, 169
Newborns
    maple syrup urine disease and, 123
    screening system for, 117, 118f,
    129
Nitrite, 5, 75–76
    infections and, 70
    test for
        clinical significance of, 75
        reaction interference with, 76
        timing of, 76
Nitroferricyanide reaction. *See* So-
    dium nitroprusside reaction
Nitroso-naphtol test, 122, 130t
Nitrous acid, 125
Nocturia, 3, 9
Normal crystals, 99
    major characteristics of, 100t
Nucleated red blood cells, 145

Occult blood, screening tests for,
    202–203
Odor, bacterial infections and, 50
Oil red O stain, 202
Oligoclonal bands, 148
Oliguria, 3, 9
Oncotic pressure, 16, 16f
1-nitroso-2-naphtol, 5-HIAA and,
    125
Ornithine, as amino acid, 125
Ortho-tolidine, 202, 203
Osmolality, 28
Osmolarity, 27–30
    clinical uses of, 29
    sweat, 184
    testing of, 47
    urine, 29
    use of in evaluating renal concen-
        tration ability, 28
Osmole, defined, 28
Osmometers, 50, 107
    clinical, 28–29
    sweat electrolytes, 184
Osmometry. *See* Reagent strips
Osmotic gradient (salt concentra-
    tion), maintenance of, 18–19
"Out of control" procedure, 108f
Oval fat bodies: epithelial cells and,
    94
Overflow disorders
    causes of, 117–118
    vs. renal, 117–119

Oxidative decarboxylation, 123
Oxygen deprivation, CSF lactate
    and, 149

PAH test, 31
p-aminohippurate (PAH), 31
Pandy test, 148
Papanicolaou's stain, 90, 94, 164
Paracentesis, 173
Parasites, 98
Parietal membrane, 173
"Pass through," 66
Passive reabsorption, 17
Passive transport, 17–18
Pasteur pipette, 142, 143
Pentagastrin: as stimulant, 194–196
Pentosuria, as inborn error of metab-
    olism, 129
Pepsin, 193
Pepsinogen, 193
Pericardial fluid, 177
    testing of, 179–180
Pericardiocentesis, 173
Peritoneal fluid, 177–179
    appearance of, 179
    testing of, 180
Peritubular capillaries, 14–15
Pernicious anemia, 196
pH, 4
    pleural fluid, 177
    semen, 162
    urinary
        clinical significance of, 60–61
        control of, 61
        crystal identification and, 98
        importance of, 60
pH-sensitive electrodes, 192
Phase microscopy, 96, 169
Phenistix, 121, 122
Phenol derivatives, 45
Phenol red, 193
Phenolphthalein, 193
Phenolsulfonphthalein, 10, 30
Phenylalanine, measuring serum lev-
    els of, 121
Phenylalanine hydroxylase, 119
Phenylalanine metabolism, 120f
Phenylalanine-tyrosine metabolism,
    119–123
Phenylalanine-tyrosine pathway,
    summary of screening tests for
    disorders of, 123
Phenylketones, 68
Phenylketonuria (PKU), 10,
    119–121
    initial screening for, 119
    keto acids and, 123
Phenylpyruvate, 119, 120f
Phenylpyruvic acid, measuring for,
    121
Phosphates, in uric alkaline crystals,
    99
Phosphatidylglycerol, as essential,
    182
Phospholipids, 181

Phthalein dyes, 68
p-hydroxyphenyllactic acid, 121
p-hydroxyphenylpyruvic acid, 121
Pia arachnoid mesothelial cells, 146
Pilocarpine iontophoresis technique,
    184
Pipettes, 142
"Pisse prophets," 1
PKU (phenylketonuria), 10
Planar hydrodynamic positioning, 60
Plaut and Silberman, on quality con-
    trol, 103
Pleocytosis, 144
Pleural fluid, 176–177
    appearance of, 176
    characteristics of in common dis-
        eases, 178t
    chemical tests on, 177
    formation of, 176
    formation and absorption of, 173,
        174f
    summary of testing, 179
Podocytes, visceral epithelial, 16f,
    17
Polarized light
    compensated, 172f
    in crystal identification, 102
    direct, 171f
    fatty casts, 97
    use of, 90
Polydipsia, 9
Polyuria, 3, 4, 9, 126
Porphobilinogen, 126, 127
Porphyrias, 126
Porphyrins
    defined, 126
    disorders of, 126–128
    occult blood test and, 203
    summary of screening tests for,
        128
Porphyrinuria, 73
    lead poisoning and, 126
    screening tests for, 126–127
Prealbumin, in CSF, 146–147
Precipitation method, 63
Pregnancy testing. *See* HCG
Procedure manual, 104
Prophobilinogen, urinary, 74
Protein, 61–64
    cerebrospinal, 146–150
    precipitation tests for, 63
    reagent strip reactions to, 62–63
    specific gravity of, 48
    urinary, summary of clinical sig-
        nificance of, 64
Protein determination test, 146–147
"Protein error of indicators," 62, 147
Protein fractions, 147–148
Proteinuria (albuminuria), 10
    benign, 62
    clinical significance of, 61–62
    orthostatic (postural), 62
    pathologic causes of, 61–62
Protoporphyrin, 71
Proximal convoluted tubule, 16f, 19,
    30

Prussian blue stain, 99
Psammoma bodies, 179
Pseudoperoxidase activity, 203
PSP (phenolsulfonphthalein), 10
PSP test, 30–31
Pyelogram, intravenous (IVP), 10, 50
Pyelonephritis, 36, 75, 96
Pyridium compounds, 45, 58, 72
Pyuria, 10, 93

Q. A. (quality assurance), 10
Q. C. (quality control), 10
qns (quantity nonsufficient), 10
Quality control
    laboratory vs. industrial, 103t
    supervision of, 103–104

RA cells, 169
Radial immunodiffusion, 148
Radiographic dye crystals, 99, 102
Radionucleotides, glomerular filtra-
        tion test and, 23
Ragocytes, 169
RBC (red blood cell), 10
RBC squares, 163
Reabsorption
    importance of assessment of, 46
    vasopressin and, 19
Reagent strip interference, 63
    Pyridium and, 58
Reagent strip reactions, 61
    blood, 69–70
    diazo, 72
    evaluating, 58
    glucose oxidase, 65
    ketones, 67–68
    leukocytes, 77
    nitrite, 75–76
    specific gravity, 76
    urinary bilirubin, 72
    urobilinogen, 74
Reagent strips, 47
    care of, 58–59
    measures specific gravity, 50
    quality control of, 58, 59
    storage of, 58
    summary of clinical testing by,
        78–79t
    technique, 55–58, 59
Reagents, quality control for, 104
Red blood cell casts, 96
Red blood cell count, 143, 163
    peritoneal fluid, 179
Red blood cells
    appearance of, 93
    disintegration of, 5
    as dysmorphic, 93
    as hypochromic, 93
    in-vitro lysis of, 43
    lysis of, 69
    significance of in urine, 92–93
    turbidity and, 45
Red stools, 200
Refractive index, principle of, 48, 49

Refractometer, 10, 47, 48–49, 107
    advantage of, 47
    calibration of, 49
    index, 47
    scale, 49f
Reiter cells, 169
Relative centrifugal force (RCF), 89
Renal, 10
Renal blood flow, 14–16
    body size and, 15–16
    tubular secretion and, 30–31
    use of radioactive hippurate to
        measure, 31
Renal calculi, 10
    analysis of, 102
    cystine and, 125
    formation of, 60
    hematuria and, 92
    presence of crystalluria and, 102
Renal concentration, 18–19, 18f
Renal dialysis, 10
Renal diseases, 32–36
    laboratory correlations in, 34–35t
    loss of tubular reabsorption capa-
        bility and, 25
Renal disorders
    causes of, 118
    vs. overflow, 117–119
Renal failure, 36
Renal failure casts, 97
Renal function
    body size and, 15–16
    measurement of, 117
    plasma creatinine measurement
        and, 23
Renal function tests, 21–30
Renal graft rejection, 94
Renal physiology, 13–21
Renal threshold, 64
    defined, 18
Renal tubular acidosis, 32
Renal tubular epithelial cells, leuko-
        cytes and, 93
Renin, function of, 17
Renin-angiotensin system, 17
Resorcinol test, 67
Respiratory distress, early delivery
        and, 181
Results, reporting of, 108–109, 108f
Reticuloendothelial system, 71
Retinopathy, diabetic, 64
Revolutions per minute (RPM), 89
Reye's syndrome, 149
Rh babies, 180
Rheumatoid arthritis, 171, 173
Ropes test, 168
Rothera test, 68

Sanfilippo's syndrome, 128
Saponin, 169
Schistosoma haematobium, 98
Screening tests
    role of laboratory in, 117
    special urinalysis, 116–131
    summary of urinary, 129–131t

Sediment, urinary, microscopic ex-
        amination, 88–89
Sediment constituents, 92–102
    control method for, 105–107
    staining reactions of, 91–92t
Sediment stains, 89–90
Semen
    appearance of, 162
    tests for presence of, 165–
        166
    viscosity, 162
    volume, 162
Semen analysis
    abnormal values for, 167t
    normal values for, 162t
    postvasectomy, 165
    testing for abnormal, 166t
Seminal fluid, 161–166
    analysis of, 161
    composition of, 161
    fructose level test for, 165
Septic arthritis, 171
Serotonin, production of, 125
Serous fluids, 173–180
    classification of, 174
    formation of, 173
    general lab procedure for, 176
    summary of testing of, 179–
        180
Serous membrane, defined, 173
Serum
    color of, 70
    osmolarity, 29
Serum gastrin levels, 193
    measurement of, 192
Serum test, carbohydrate malabsorp-
        tion or intolerance, 204
SG (specific gravity), 10
"Shake" test, 183
Silver-nitroprusside test, 126
Simulated spinal fluid (SSF) proce-
        dure, 153
Single radial immunodiffusion arthri-
        tis diagnosis, 173
Slow vibration, 170
Sodium, measurement of, 184
Sodium nitroprusside test, 122
    interference in, 68
Sound-wave frequency, specific
        gravity and, 60
Specialized G cells, 193
Specific gravity (Sp. gr. or SG), 10,
        46–50
    ADH and, 46
    clinical correlations of, 49–50
    defined, 46
    falling drop method of measuring,
        59
    in Fishberg test, 27
    as measured by urinometer, 28
    Mosenthal test, 27
    Multistix and, 76
    reabsorption and, 46
    sound-wave frequency and, 60
    urinary, summary of clinical sig-
        nificance of, 77

Specimens, urinary
appearance of, terms used, 45
catheterized, 8–9
clarity of, 46
collection of, 4
fasting, 7
first morning, 7
glucose tolerance test, 8
midstream clean-catch, 9
normal, appearance of, 45
pediatric, 9
policies on handling, 4, 104
policy for handling mislabeled, 106t
postvasectomy, 162
preservation of, 4, 5t
random, 7
suprapubic aspiration, 9
24-hour (timed), 8
2-hour postprandial, 8
types of, 6–9, 7t
unique characteristics of, 2
Spectrophotometry, 63
amniotic fluid, 181
bilirubin scans, 182f
homogentisic acid and, 122
use of in PSP test, 31
Sperm agglutinating antibodies, test for, 165
Sperm count, as measure of fertility, 163
Sperm morphology
abnormal, 165f
evaluation of, 164–166
Sperm motility, laboratory evaluation of, 163–164
Sperm viability, tests for, 165
Spermatids, 164
Spermatozoa, 98, 161
Sp. Gr. (specific gravity), 10
Sphingomyelin, measurement of, 182
Spina bifida, 183
Squamous epithelial cells, 45, 94
Staphylococcus, 173
Steatorrhea, 200–201
causes of, 202
diagnosis of, 202
fecal fats and, 202
Sternheimer-Malbin stain, 90
glitter cells and, 93
hyaline casts, 96
renal tubular epithelial cells and, 94
Stools
abnormalities in, 201
major characteristics of, 201t
Streptococci, as origin of acute glomerulonephritis, 32, 33
Streptococcus, 173
Streptococcus pneumoniae, 152
Strontium peroxide, 203
Sudan III staining
fatty casts, 97
fecal fats, 202
pleural fluid, 176

renal tubular cells, 94
Sudan IV, 202
Sulfonamides, 99, 102
Sulfosalicylic acid test, 63
Sulkowitch's reagent, 129
Sulkowitch's test, 129
Sweat, 183–184
Sweat electrolytes
method for measuring, 184
vs. sweat osmolarity, 184
Sweat osmolarity, sweat electrolytes and, 184
Sweat specimens, collection and handling of, 184
Synovial fluid, 166–173
appearance of, 167
cells and inclusions in, 170t
chemical composition of, 166
in chemical laboratory, 172
collection of, 167
function of, 166
in hematology laboratory, 167–171
in microbiology laboratory, 172–173
purpose of analysis of, 167
in serology laboratory, 173
viscosity of, 168
Synovial fluid protein, measurement of, 171
Syphilis, 152
Systemic lupus erythematosus, 32, 33

Tamm-Horsfield protein, 61, 95
Tartaric acid, 203
"Tau" (transferrin fraction), 147
Temperature, urinometer and, 47
Tetramethylbenzidine, 69–70
Thoracentesis, 173
"Thorny apples," 99
Titratable acidity, urinary ammonia and, 32
Titration procedures
current, 193–194
old, 193
Titration results, 193–194
Tm (maximal reabsorptive capacity), 18
TNTC (too numerous to count), 10, 89
Toilet bowl cleaner, 203
Tolbutamide (ingestion), 63
"Too numerous to count" (TNTC), 10, 89
Töpfer's reagent, 193
Total cell count, 142
Tract infections, 60–61
Transferrin, 147
Transudates
classification of, 175t
defined, 174
laboratory differentiation of exudates and, 175t
Traumatic collection, 140–141

"Traumatic tap," 140
Trichomonas vaginalis, 98
Trichoracetic acid. *See* Fouchet's reagent
Triglycerides, 202
Triple phosphate, 99
Trypsin, screening test for, 204
Tryptophan metabolism, 124f, 124–125
Tube tests, for ketone measurement, 68
Tubercular meningitis, 146
antibody stains and, 151
symptoms of, 149
Tuberculosis, 176
Tubular disorders, protein levels of, 62
Tubular necrosis, 94
Tubular reabsorption, 17–18
cellular mechanisms in, 17–18
tests, 25–30
Tubular secretion, 19–21
renal blood flow tests and, 30–31
Turbidimetric method, measuring CSF protein, 147
Turbidity, 5
causes of, 45–46
laboratory correlations in, 46t
nonpathogenic causes of, 46
in pleural fluid, 176
in synovial fluid, 167
Turbidity production, technique of, 147
2,4-dinitrophenyl-hydrazine (DNAH) reaction, 123
Tyrosine crystals, 99, 102
Tyrosine metabolism, 120f
Tyrosinemia, 121
transitory, 121
Tyrosyluria, 119, 121–122

UA (routine urinalysis), 10
Ulcerative colitis, 201
Urea
defined, 2
use of as test substance, 23
Urea molecules, 47
Uremia, 10
-uria, 10
Uric acid, 2
Urinalysis
automation in, 59–60
correlations in, 90t
defined, 10
history of, 1–2
importance of, 1–2
panic values, 110t
as part of routine physical exam, 2
quality assurance in, 87–110
special screening tests for, 116–131
standardization report on, 109t
as valuable metabolic screening procedure, 2
Urinalysis laboratory

responsibility of, 117
screening tests and, 117
Urine
  abnormal metabolic substances in, 117–118, 117t
  characteristics of, 1
  chemical examination of, 54–79
  composition of, 2
  density (specific gravity) of, 23, 27f
  formation of, 2
  major chemical substances in, 2, 3t
  microscopic examination of, 87–110
  normal ranges of, 105t
  physical examination of, 42–53
  screening of for metabolic disease, 118f
  unpreserved
    changes in, 4–5, 5–6t
  volume of, 3
Urine concentration, body's state of hydration and, 25
Urine culture
  after nitrite test, 76
  as primary test for infection, 75
Urine specimen. See Specimens
Urine stasis, 97
Urine turbidity. See Turbidity
Urinometer, 10, 47–48, 47f, 107
  disadvantage of, 47
  as measure of specific gravity, 28, 47
  temperature and, 47

Urobilin, 71, 73, 200
Urobilinogen, 5, 71, 73–74
Urochrome, 43
Uroerythrin, 45
Urologist, 10
Urology, 10
Uroscopy, art of, 1–2

Vaginal moniliasis, 98
Vagus nerve, 196
Valine, as amino acid, 123
Valinemia, 121
Van de Kamer titration, 203
Vapor pressure osmometer, 29
Vasa recta, 15
Vasopressin, 19
VDRL (Venereal Disease Research Laboratories) procedure, 152
Viral meningitis, 146
  LD isoenzymes and, 150
  symptoms of, 149
Visceral membrane, 173
Vitamin C, 203
Volume, urine, factors that influence, 3

Water, as major body constituent, 3
Watson urobilinogen test, 74
Watson-Schwartz Differentiation Test, 74
  prophyrinuria and, 126
Waxy casts, 97

WBC (white blood cell), 10
Webster Sweat Collection System, 184
Whatman no. 1 filter paper, 128
White blood cell casts, 96
White blood cell count, 142, 143
  peritoneal fluid, 179
White blood cell squares, 163
White blood cells, 93–94
  appearance of, 93
  artificially added, 143
  in feces, 201
  spermatids and, 164
  turbidity and, 45
Wollaston, William Hyde, 125
Wright's stain
  CSF specimen, 143
  feces, 201
  red blood cells, 93

Xanthochromia, 139–140
Xanthochromic supernatant, 141

Yeast cells, 93, 98
Yellow foam, bilirubin and, 43
Yellow IRIS, 59
  advantage of, 60

Zollinger-Ellison syndrome, 192
  defined, 194
Zymogen chief cells, 193